ABBREVIATIONS

DRUG OR DRUG CLASS	FULL NAME
α-1 Blockers	Alpha-1 Adrenergic Blockers
β-Blockers	Beta-Adrenergic Blockers
ACE Inhibitors	Angiotensin Converting Enzyme Inhibitors
BZD	Benzodiazepines
CCB	Calcium Channel Blockers
CCB, dihydropyridine	Dihydropyridine Calcium Channel Blockers
FLQ	Fluoroquinolones
HCTZ	Hydrochlorothiazide
LMWH	Low Molecular Weight Heparins
MAOIs	Monoamine Oxidase Inhibitors
NSAIDs	Nonsteroidal Anti-inflammatory Drugs
SSRIs	Selective Serotonin Reuptake Inhibitors
TCAs	Tricyclic Antidepressants

Acetaminophen/codeine	Tylenol w/Codeine #3, Tylenol w/Codeine #4	2, 64
Acyclovir	Zovirax	2
Albuterol	Accuneb, ProAir HFA, Proventil, Proventil HFA, Ventolin, Ventolin HFA	3
Albuterol sulfate/ipratropium bromide	Combivent	3, 152
Alendronate sodium	Fosamax	3
Allopurinol	Zyloprim	3
Alprazolam	Niravam, Xanax, Xanax XR	4
Amitriptyline	Elavil	7
Amlodipine besylate	Norvasc	13
Amlodipine besylate/benazepril HCl	Lotrel	13, 27
Amoxicillin	Amoxil, Dispermox, Trimox	14
Amoxicillin/clavulanate potassium	Augmentin, Augmentin XR, Augmentin ES-600	14
Amphetamine salt combination	Adderall, Adderall XR	15
Aripiprazole	Abilify, Abilify Discmelt	16
Aspirin	Bayer Aspirin, Ecotrin, Halfprin, St. Joseph's	16
Atenolol	Tenormin	20
Atenolol/chlorthalidone	Tenoretic	20, 45
Atomoxetine HCl	Strattera	21

Atorvastatin calcium	Lipitor	23
Azelastine HCl	Astelin	26
Azithromycin	AzaSite, Zithromax, Zmax	26
Benazepril HCl	Lotensin	27
Bisoprolol/hydrochlorothiazide	Ziac	31, 142
Budesonide	Rhinocort Aqua, Entocort EC, Pulmicort	32
Buprenorphine HCl/naloxone HCl	Suboxone	33, 211
Bupropion	Budeprion SR, Budeprion XL, Wellbutrin, Wellbutrin SR, Wellbutrin XL, Zyban	35
Buspirone HCl	Buspar, Vanspar	37
Butalbital/caffeine/acetaminophen	Fioricet	39, 40, 2
Carisoprodol	Soma	41
Carvedilol phosphate	Coreg, Coreg CR	41
Cefuroxime axetil	Ceftin	43
Celecoxib	Celebrex	43
Cephalexin	Keflex	45
Cetirizine HCl/pseudoephedrine HCl	Zyrtec-D	267
Ciprofloxacin HCl	Cipro, Cipro XR, Ciloxan, Proquin XR	47
Citalopram HBr	Celexa	49

Clarithromycin	Biaxin, Biaxin XL	54
Clindamycin systemic	Cleocin	59
Clonazepam	Klonopin	59
Clonidine	Catapres, Catapres TTS	60
Clopidogrel bisulfate	Plavix	62
Clotrimazole/betamethasone	Lotrisone	63, 29
Colchicine*	Colchicine*	65
Cyclobenzaprine	Flexeril	67
Desogestrel/ethinyl estradiol	Apri, Cyclessa, Desogen, Kariva, Mircette, Ortho-Cept, Velivet	67, 96
Diazepam	Valium, Diastat	68
Diclofenac	Flector, Solaraze, Voltaren, Voltaren XR	70
Dicyclomine HCl	Bentyl	73
Digoxin	Lanoxin, Digitek	73
Diltiazem CD	Cardizem, Cardizem CD, Cardizem LA, Cardizem SR, Cartia XT, Dilacor XR, Dilt-CD, Taztia XT, Tiazac	79
Divalproex sodium (valproic acid)	Depakote, Depakote ER	311
Doxazosin	Cardura, Cardura XL	84
Doxycycline	Monodox, Adoxa, Oracea, Vibramycin	84

Drospirenone/ethinyl estradiol	Yasmin, YAZ	85, 96
Duloxetine HCl	Cymbalta	86
Dutasteride	Avodart	89
Enalapril*	Enalapril*	90
Escitalopram oxalate	Lexapro	92
Esomeprazole sodium	Nexium	95
Estradiol	Alora, Climara, Estrace, Estraderm, Estrasorb, Femring, Gynodiol, Menostar, Vivelle, Vivelle-Dot	95
Estrogen, conjugated	Premarin	66
Eszopiclone	Lunesta	96
Etodolac	Lodine, Lodine XL	100
Etonogestrel/ethinyl estradiol	NuvaRing	103, 96
Ezetimibe	Zetia	105
Famotidine	Pepcid	105
Felodipine	Plendil, Plendil ER	106
Fenofibrate	Tricor	108
Fentanyl	Actiq, Duragesic, Ionsys, Sublimaze	109
Ferrous sulfate (iron)	Slow Fe	153
Fexofenadine	Allegra	114

Fexofenadine/pseudoephedrine	**Allegra-D 12 Hour, Allegra-D 24 Hour**	114, 267
Finasteride	**Propecia, Proscar**	115
Fluconazole	**Diflucan**	115
Fluoxetine	**Prozac, Sarafem**	120
Fluticasone	**Cutivate, Flonase, Flovent, Flovent HFA, Veramyst**	127
Fluticasone propionate/salmeterol	**Advair Diskus, Advair HFA**	127, 279
Folic acid*	**Folic acid***	127
Fosinopril sodium	**Monopril**	127
Furosemide	**Lasix**	130
Gabapentin	**Neurontin**	133
Gemfibrozil	**Lopid**	133
Glimepiride	**Amaryl**	135
Glipizide	**Glucotrol, Glucotrol XL**	137
Glyburide	**Diabeta, Glynase, Micronase**	139
Glyburide/metformin HCl	**Glucovance**	139, 188
Hydrochlorothiazide*	**hydrochlorothiazide***	142
Hydrocodone polistirex/ chlorpheniramine polistirex	**Tussionex**	146

Hydrocodone/acetaminophen	Allay, Anexsia, Lortab, Norcet, Norco, Vicodin, Vicodin ES, Vicodin HP, Zydone	146, 2
Hydroxychloroquine	Plaquenil	147
Ibandronate sodium	Boniva	147
Ibuprofen	Motrin, Advil	147
Insulin glargine, human	Lantus	150
Insulin lispro	Humalog	151
Insulin, human isophane	Humulin N	150
Irbesartan	Avapro	152
Irbesartan/hydrochlorothiazide	Avalide	152, 142
Ketoconazole	Nizoral, Xolegel	155
Lamotrigine	Lamictal, Lamictal CD	163
Lansoprazole	Prevacid, Prevacid IV, Prevacid Solutab	164
Latanoprost	Xalatan	166
Levetiracetam	Keppra	166
Levofloxacin	Levaquin, Quixin	166
Levonorgestrel/estradiol	Climara Pro	168, 95
Levonorgestrel/ethinyl estradiol	Alesse, Aviane, Enpresse, Lessina, Levlite, Levora, Lybrel, Nordette, Portia, Quasense, Seasonale, Seasonique, Triphasil, Trivora	168, 96

Levothyroxine	Levoxyl, Synthroid, Levothroid, Unithroid	170
Lidocaine	Lidoderm, Xylocaine	172
Lisinopril	Prinivil, Zestril	174
Lisinopril/hydrochlorothiazide	Prinizide, Zestoretic	174, 142
Lithium carbonate	Lithobid, Eskalith, Eskalith CR	175
Lorazepam	Ativan	182
Losartan potassium	Cozaar	182
Losartan potassium/hydrochlorothiazide	Hyzaar	182, 142
Lovastatin	Mevacor, Altroprev	184
Meloxicam	Mobic	186
Metaxalone	Skelaxin	188
Metformin	Fortamet, Glucophage, Glucophage XR, Glumetza, Riomet	188
Methocarbamol	Robaxin	191
Methotrexate	Trexall	191
Methylphenidate	Concerta, Daytrana, Metadate CD, Metadate ER, Methylin, Methylin ER, Ritalin, Ritalin LA, Ritalin SR	195
Methylprednisolone	Depo-Medrol, Medrol, Solu-Medrol	195
Metoclopramide	Reglan	198

Metoprolol succinate	Toprol XL	199
Metoprolol tartrate	Lopressor	199
Metoprolol tartrate/hydrochlorothiazide	Lopressor HCT	199, 142
Metronidazole	Flagyl, Flagyl ER, Metrocream, Metrogel, Metrogel-Vaginal, Metrolotion, Noritate, Vandazole	202
Minocycline	Dynacin, Minocin, Solodyn	204
Mirtazapine	Remeron, Remeron Soltab	205
Mometasone furoate monohydrate	Nasonex	205
Montelukast sodium	Singulair	205
Morphine sulfate	Avinza, Astramorph PF, Depodur, Duramorph PF, Infumorph, Kadian, MS Contin, MS IR, Oramorph SR, Roxanol	206
Moxifloxacin HCl	Avelox, Vigamox	207
Nabumetone	Relafen	209
Naproxen	Anaprox, Anaprox DS, Naprelan, Naprosyn, EC Naprosyn	211
Niacin	Niaspan	213
Nifedipine	Adalat, Adalat CC, Procardia, Procardia XL	214
Nitrofurantoin	Macrobid, Furadantin, Macrodantin	216
Nitroglycerin	NitroStat, NitroQuick	217
Norelgestromin/ethinyl estradiol	Ortho Evra	217, 96

Norethindrone acetate/estradiol	Activella, CombiPatch	217, 95
Norethindrone acetate/ethinyl estradiol	Estrostep FE, femhrt, Junel, Junel FE, Loestrin, Loestrin FE, Microgestin FE, Ovcon, Tri-Norinyl	217, 96
Norgestimate/ethinyl estradiol	Ortho Cyclen, Ortho Tri-Cylen, Ortho Tri-Cyclen Lo, Previfem, Sprintec, Tri-Previfem, Tri-Sprintec	220, 96
Nortriptyline	Pamelor	225
Olanzapine	Zyprexa	229
Omeprazole	Prilosec	230
Oseltamivir phosphate	Tamiflu	232
Oxycodone	Oxycontin, Roxicodone, Oxy IR	232
Oxycodone HCl/acetaminophen	Endocet, Percocet, Roxicet	232, 2
Pantoprazole sodium	Protonix	234
Paroxetine	Paxil, Paxil CR, Pexeva	234
Penicillin v potassium	Pen-VK, Veetids	242
Phenobarbital*	Phenobarbital*	242
Phentermine	Adipex-P	246
Phenytoin sodium	Dilantin, Phenytek	246
Pioglitazone HCl	Actos	256
Potassium chloride	K-Lor, K-Tab, K-Dur, Klor-Con, Micro-K	257

Pravastatin sodium	Pravachol	258
Prednisolone sodium phosphate	Orapred, Orapred ODT, Pediapred	260
Prednisone*	Prednisone*	262
Promethazine	Phenergan	264
Promethazine/codeine	Phenergan w/Codeine	264, 64
Propoxyphene napsylate/ acetaminophen	Darvocet A500, Darvocet-N	266, 2
Quetiapine fumarate	Seroquel, Seroquel XR	268
Quinapril	Accupril	269
Quinine sulfate*	Quinine sulfate*	271
Rabeprazole sodium	Aciphex	272
Ramipril	Altace	272
Ranitidine HCl	Zantac	274
Risedronate sodium	Actonel	275
Risperidone	Risperdal, Risperdal Consta	275
Ropinirole HCl	Requip	277
Rosiglitazone maleate	Avandia	277
Rosuvastatin calcium	Crestor	278
Sertraline HCl	Zoloft	280

Sildenafil citrate	Revatio, Viagra	287
Simvastatin	Zocor	289
Simvastatin/ezetimibe	Vytorin	289, 105
Sitagliptin	Januvia	293
Sitagliptin/metformin	Janumet	293, 188
Spironolactone	Aldactone	293
Sumatriptan	Imitrex	296
Tadalafil	Cialis	297
Tamsulosin HCl	Flomax	298
Temazepam	Restoril	298
Terazosin	Hytrin	299
Tizanidine HCl	Zanaflex	300
Tolterodine tartrate	Detrol, Detrol LA	300
Topiramate	Topamax, Topamax Sprinkle Capsules	301
Tramadol	Ultram, Ultram ER	302
Tramadol HCl/acetaminophen	Ultracet	302, 2
Trazodone HCl	Desyrel	303
Triamcinolone acetonide	Kenalog, Nasacort AQ, Nasacort HFA, Azmacort, Oracort, Oralone, Triacet	305

Triamterene/hydrochlorothiazide	Dyazide, Maxzide	307, 142
Trimethoprim/sulfamethoxazole	Bactrim, Bactrim DS, Cotrim, Cotrim DS, Septra, Septra DS	309, 294
Valacyclovir HCI	Valtrex	311
Valsartan	Diovan	313
Valsartan/hydrochlorothiazide	Diovan HCT	313, 142
Varenicline	Chantix	314
Venlafaxine HCI	Effexor, Effexor XR	314
Verapamil	Calan, Covera-HS, Isoptin, Isoptin SR, Verelan, Veralan PM	318
Warfarin	Coumadin, Jantoven	322
Zolpidem tartrate	Ambien, Ambien CR	333

A-to-Z Generic Drugs

ACETAMINOPHEN

acenocoumarol	2	3	2	May result in potentiation of anticoagulant effect.
cabbage	1	3	2	May result in decreased acetaminophen effectiveness.
carbamazepine	2	3	2	May result in increased risk of acetaminophen hepatotoxicity.
ethanol	2	2	2	May result in increased risk of hepatotoxicity.
isoniazid	2	3	2	May result in increased risk of hepatotoxicity.
phenytoin	2	3	2	May result in decreased acetaminophen effectiveness and an increased risk of hepatotoxicity.
uric acid measurement	1	3	2	May result in falsely increased serum uric acid levels due to assay interference with the phosphotungstate reduction method.
warfarin	2	3	1	May result in increased risk of bleeding.
zidovudine	2	3	2	May result in neutropenia; acetaminophen toxicity (hepatotoxicity).

ACYCLOVIR

fosphenytoin	2	3	2	May result in decreased phenytoin plasma concentrations and potential increased seizure activity.
phenytoin	2	3	2	May result in decreased phenytoin plasma concentrations and potential increased seizure activity.

valproic acid	2	3	2	May result in decreased valproic acid plasma concentrations and potential increased seizure activity.

ALBUTEROL

atomoxetine	0	2	2	May result in increase in heart rate and blood pressure.
MAOIs (*clorgyline, iproniazide, isocarboxazid, moclobemide, nialamide, pargyline, phenelzine, procarbazine, selegiline, toloxatone, tranylcypromine*)	2	2	2	May result in increased risk of tachycardia, agitation, or hypomania.

ALENDRONATE

dairy food	1	3	2	May result in reduced alendronate exposure.

ALLOPURINOL

aluminum hydroxide	2	3	2	May result in decreased allopurinol effectiveness.
azathioprine	2	2	1	May result in azathioprine toxicity (nausea, vomiting, leukopenia, anemia).
captopril	2	2	2	May result in hypersensitivity reactions (Stevens-Johnson syndrome, skin eruptions).
cyclophosphamide	2	2	2	May result in cyclophosphamide toxicity (bone marrow suppression, nausea, vomiting).
cyclosporine	2	3	2	May result in increased risk of cyclosporine toxicity (renal dysfunction, cholestasis, paresthesias).

ONSET: 0 - NOT SPECIFIED 1 - RAPID 2 - DELAYED   SEVERITY: 1 - CONTRAINDICATED 2 - MAJOR 3 - MODERATE

didanosine	1	3	2	May result in increased serum concentrations of didanosine.
enalapril maleate	1	2	2	May result in hypersensitivity reactions (Stevens-Johnson syndrome, skin eruptions, anaphylactic coronary spasm).
enalaprilat	1	2	2	May result in hypersensitivity reactions (Stevens-Johnson syndrome, skin eruptions, anaphylactic coronary spasm).
mercaptopurine	2	2	2	May result in mercaptopurine toxicity (bone marrow suppression, nausea, vomiting).
phenprocoumon	2	3	2	May result in increased risk of bleeding.
vidarabine	2	3	2	May result in neurotoxicity, tremors, impaired cognitive function.
warfarin	2	3	2	May result in increased risk of bleeding.
ALPRAZOLAM				
amprenavir	2	3	2	May result in increased risk of alprazolam toxicity (excessive sedation, confusion).
aprepitant	1	3	2	May result in increased systemic exposure of BZD.
Barbiturates (*amobarbital, aprobarbital, butabarbital, butalbital, mephobarbital, methohexital, pentobarbital, phenobarbital, primidone, secobarbital, thiopental*)	0	2	2	May result in additive respiratory depression.

carbamazepine	2	3	2	May result in decreased alprazolam effectiveness.
cimetidine	1	3	2	May result in increased risk of alprazolam toxicity (CNS depression).
clarithromycin	2	3	2	May result in increased BZD toxicity (CNS depression, ataxia, lethargy).
Contraceptives, Combination (*desogestrel, drospirenone, estradiol cypionate, ethinyl estradiol, ethynodiol diacetate, etonogestrel, levonorgestrel, medroxyprogesterone acetate, mestranol, norelgestromin, norethindrone, norgestimate, norgestrel*)	2	3	2	May result in increased risk of alprazolam toxicity (CNS depression, hypotension).
desipramine	0	3	2	May result in increased desipramine plasma concentrations.
digoxin	2	2	2	May result in digoxin toxicity (nausea, vomiting, arrhythmias).
erythromycin	2	3	2	May result in increased BZD toxicity (CNS depression, ataxia, lethargy).
fluoxetine	1	3	2	May result in increased risk of alprazolam toxicity (somnolence, dizziness, ataxia, slurred speech, hypotension, psychomotor impairment).
fosamprenavir	2	3	2	May result in increased risk of alprazolam toxicity (excessive sedation, confusion, respiratory depression).

ONSET: 0 - NOT SPECIFIED 1 - RAPID 2 - DELAYED   SEVERITY: 1 - CONTRAINDICATED 2 - MAJOR 3 - MODERATE

imipramine	0	3	2	May result in increased imipramine plasma concentrations.
itraconazole	0	1	1	May result in increased alprazolam concentrations and potential alprazolam toxicity (excessive sedation and prolonged hypnotic effects).
kava	2	3	2	May result in increased CNS depression.
ketoconazole	0	1	1	May result in increased alprazolam concentrations and potential alprazolam toxicity (excessive sedation and prolonged hypnotic effects).
nefazodone	1	3	2	May result in psychomotor impairment and sedation.
Opioid Analgesics (*alfentanil, anileridine, codeine, fentanyl, hydrocodone, hydromorphone, levorphanol, meperidine, morphine, morphine sulfate, oxycodone, oxymorphone, propoxyphene, remifentanyl, sufentanil*)	0	2	2	May result in additive respiratory depression.
rifapentine	2	3	2	May result in reduced diazepam plasma concentrations and effectiveness.
ritonavir	2	3	2	May result in increased plasma concentrations of alprazolam and enhanced alprazolam effects.
roxithromycin	2	3	2	May result in increased BZD toxicity (CNS depression, ataxia, lethargy).

sertraline	1	3	2	May result in increased risk of psychomotor impairment and sedation.
St. John's wort	2	3	2	May result in reduced BZD effectiveness.
theophylline	1	3	2	May result in decreased BZD effectiveness.
troleandomycin	2	3	2	May result in increased BZD toxicity (CNS depression, ataxia, lethargy).
AMITRIPTYLINE				
acenocoumarol	2	3	2	May result in increased risk of bleeding.
amprenavir	2	2	2	May result in increased tricyclic serum concentrations and potential toxicity (anticholinergic effects, sedation, confusion, cardiac arrhythmias).
Antiarrhythmic Agents, Class IA (*ajmaline, disopyramide, hydroquinidine, pirmenol, prajmaline, procainamide*)	0	2	2	May result in increased risk of cardiotoxicity (QT prolongation, torsades de pointes, cardiac arrest).
arbutamine	1	3	2	May result in unreliable arbutamine test results.
atomoxetine	0	3	2	May result in increased atomoxetine steady-state plasma concentrations.
bethanidine	1	3	2	May result in decreased antihypertensive effectiveness.
carbamazepine	2	3	2	May result in decreased amitriptyline effectiveness.

ONSET: 0 – NOT SPECIFIED, 1 – RAPID, 2 – DELAYED SEVERITY: 1 – CONTRAINDICATED, 2 – MAJOR, 3 – MODERATE

cimetidine	2	3	2	May result in amitriptyline toxicity (dry mouth, blurred vision, urinary retention).
cinacalcet	0	3	2	May result in increased amitriptyline serum concentrations and potential toxicity (anticholinergic effects, sedation, confusion, cardiac arrhythmias).
clonidine	2	2	2	May result in decreased antihypertensive effectiveness.
clorgyline	2	1	1	May result in neurotoxicity, seizures, or serotonin syndrome (hypertension, hyperthermia, myoclonus, mental status changes).
diazepam	1	3	2	May result in psychomotor deficits (decreased reaction time, decreased vigilance).
dicumarol	2	3	2	May result in increased risk of bleeding.
duloxetine	0	3	2	May result in increased tricyclic antidepressant serum concentrations and potential toxicity (anticholinergic effects, sedation, confusion, cardiac arrhythmias).
enflurane	0	2	2	May result in increased risk of cardiotoxicity (QT prolongation, torsades de pointes, cardiac arrest) and an increased risk of seizure activity.
ethanol	1	3	2	May result in enhanced CNS depression and impairment of motor skills.

fluconazole	2	2	2	May result in increased risk of amitriptyline toxicity and an increased risk of cardiotoxicity (QT prolongation, torsades de pointes, cardiac arrest).
fluoxetine	0	2	2	May result in tricyclic antidepressant toxicity (dry mouth, urinary retention, sedation) and an increased risk of cardiotoxicity (QT prolongation, torsades de pointes, cardiac arrest).
fluvoxamine	2	3	2	May result in amitriptyline toxicity (dry mouth, urinary retention, sedation).
fosamprenavir	2	2	2	May result in increased tricyclic agent serum concentrations and potential toxicity (anticholinergic effects, sedation, confusion, cardiac arrhythmias).
furazolidone	2	1	2	May result in neurotoxicity, seizures, or serotonin syndrome (hypertension, hyperthermia, myoclonus, mental status changes).
galantamine	0	3	2	May result in increased galantamine plasma concentrations.
grepafloxacin	2	1	2	May result in increased risk of cardiotoxicity (QT prolongation, torsades de pointes, cardiac arrest).
guanethidine	2	3	2	May result in decreased antihypertensive effectiveness.
halofantrine	2	2	2	May result in increased risk of cardiotoxicity (QT prolongation, torsades de pointes, cardiac arrest).

ONSET: 0 - NOT SPECIFIED, 1 - RAPID, 2 - DELAYED   SEVERITY: 1 - CONTRAINDICATED, 2 - MAJOR, 3 - MODERATE

iproniazid	2	1	2	May result in neurotoxicity, seizures, or serotonin syndrome (hypertension, hyperthermia, myoclonus, mental status changes).
isocarboxazid	2	1	1	May result in neurotoxicity, seizures, or serotonin syndrome (hypertension, hyperthermia, myoclonus, mental status changes).
linezolid	0	2	2	May result in increased risk of serotonin syndrome (hyperthermia, hyperreflexia, myoclonus, mental status changes).
moclobemide	2	1	2	May result in neurotoxicity, seizures, or serotonin syndrome (hypertension, hyperthermia, myoclonus, mental status changes).
nefazodone	1	2	2	May result in increased risk of serotonin syndrome (hypertension, hyperthermia, myoclonus, mental status changes).
nefopam	1	2	2	May result in increased risk of seizures.
nialamide	2	1	2	May result in neurotoxicity, seizures, or serotonin syndrome (hypertension, hyperthermia, myoclonus, mental status changes).
pargyline	2	1	2	May result in neurotoxicity, seizures, or serotonin syndrome (hypertension, hyperthermia, myoclonus, mental status changes).

paroxetine	2	3	2	May result in amitriptyline toxicity (dry mouth, sedation, urinary retention).
phenelzine	2	1	1	May result in neurotoxicity, seizures, or serotonin syndrome (hypertension, hyperthermia, myoclonus, mental status changes).
Phenothiazines (*prochlorperazine, trifluoperazine*)	1	2	2	May result in increased risk of cardiotoxicity (QT prolongation, torsades de pointes, cardiac arrest).
phenprocoumon	2	3	2	May result in increased risk of bleeding.
phenytoin	2	3	2	May result in increased risk of phenytoin toxicity (ataxia, hyperreflexia, nystagmus, tremor).
rifapentine	2	3	2	May result in decreased amitriptyline efficacy.
ritonavir	2	3	2	May result in increased amitriptyline serum concentrations and potential toxicity (anticholinergic effects, sedation, confusion, cardiac arrhythmias).
s-adenosylmethionine	2	3	2	May result in increased risk of serotonin syndrome (hypertension, hyperthermia, myoclonus, mental status changes).
selegiline	1	1	1	May result in neurotoxicity, seizures, or serotonin syndrome (hypertension, hyperthermia, myoclonus, mental status changes).

ONSET: 0 = NOT SPECIFIED, 1 = RAPID, 2 = DELAYED   SEVERITY: 1 = CONTRAINDICATED, 2 = MAJOR, 3 = MODERATE

sertraline	2	2	2	May result in elevated amitriptyline serum levels or possible serotonin syndrome (hypertension, hyperthermia, myoclonus, mental status changes).
St. John's wort	2	3	2	May result in decreased effectiveness of amitriptyline and possible increased risk of serotonin syndrome (hypertension, hyperthermia, myoclonus, mental status changes).
sulfamethoxazole	0	2	2	May result in increased risk of cardiotoxicity (QT prolongation, torsades de pointes, cardiac arrest).
Sympathomimetics, Direct Acting (*epinephrine, etilefrine, methoxamine, midodrine, norepinephrine, oxilofrine, phenylephrine*)	1	2	2	May result in hypertension, cardiac arrhythmias, and tachycardia.
toloxatone	2	1	2	May result in neurotoxicity, seizures, or serotonin syndrome (hypertension, hyperthermia, myoclonus, mental status changes).
tranylcypromine	2	1	1	May result in neurotoxicity, seizures, or serotonin syndrome (hypertension, hyperthermia, myoclonus, mental status changes).
trimethoprim	0	2	2	May result in increased risk of cardiotoxicity (QT prolongation, torsades de pointes, cardiac arrest).
warfarin	2	3	2	May result in increased risk of bleeding.

AMLODIPINE

Drug				Effect
amiodarone	1	2	2	May result in bradycardia, atrioventricular block and/or sinus arrest.
β-Blockers (*acebutolol, alprenolol, atenolol, betaxolol, bevantolol, bisoprolol, bucindolol, carteolol, carvedilol, celiprolol, dilevalol, esmolol, labetalol, levobunolol, mepindolol, metipranolol, metoprolol, nadolol, nebivolol, oxprenolol, penbutolol, pindolol, propranolol, sotalol, talinolol, tertatolol, timolol*)	1	3	2	May result in hypotension and/or bradycardia.
conivaptan	0	3	2	May result in increased amlodipine exposure.
dalfopristin	2	3	2	May result in increased risk of amlodipine toxicity (dizziness, hypotension, flushing, headache, peripheral edema).
fentanyl	1	2	2	May result in severe hypotension.
fluconazole	2	3	2	May result in increased amlodipine serum concentrations and toxicity (dizziness, hypotension, flushing, headache, peripheral edema).
indinavir	0	3	2	May result in increased plasma concentrations of CCB.

ONSET: 0 - NOT SPECIFIE   , RAPID, 2 - DELAYED   SEVERITY: 1 - CONTRAINDICATED, 2 - MAJOR, 3 - MODERATE

itraconazole	2	3	2	May result in increased amlodipine serum concentrations and toxicity (dizziness, hypotension, flushing, headache, peripheral edema).
ketoconazole	2	3	2	May result in increased amlodipine serum concentrations and toxicity (dizziness, hypotension, flushing, headache, peripheral edema).
quinupristin	2	3	2	May result in increased risk of amlodipine toxicity (dizziness, hypotension, flushing, headache, peripheral edema).
rifapentine	2	3	2	May result in decreased CCB effectiveness.
ritonavir	2	3	2	May result in increased amlodipine serum concentrations and potential toxicity (dizziness, headache, flushing, peripheral edema, hypotension, cardiac arrhythmias).
saquinavir	1	3	2	May result in increased risk of amlodipine toxicity (dizziness, headache, flushing, peripheral edema, hypotension, cardiac arrhythmias).
St. John's wort	2	3	2	May result in reduced bioavailability of CCB.
voriconazole	0	3	2	May result in increased plasma concentrations of CCB.
AMOXICILLIN				
acenocoumarol	0	3	2	May result in increased risk of bleeding.

Contraceptives, Combination (*ethinyl estradiol, mestranol, norelgestromin, norethindrone, norgestrel*)	2	3	2	May result in decreased contraceptive effectiveness.
khat	1	3	2	May result in reduced effectiveness of amoxicillin.
methotrexate	2	2	2	May result in methotrexate toxicity.
probenecid	2	3	2	May result in prolonged and increased amoxicillin serum concentrations.
warfarin	0	3	2	May result in increased risk of bleeding.
AMPHETAMINE				
clorgyline	1	1	1	May result in hypertensive crisis (headache, hyperpyrexia, hypertension).
guanethidine	1	3	2	May result in decreased guanethidine effectiveness.
iproniazid	1	1	2	May result in hypertensive crisis (headache, hyperpyrexia, hypertension).
isocarboxazid	1	1	1	May result in hypertensive crisis (headache, hyperpyrexia, hypertension).
nialamide	1	1	2	May result in hypertensive crisis (headache, hyperpyrexia, hypertension).
pargyline	1	1	2	May result in hypertensive crisis (headache, hyperpyrexia, hypertension).

ONSET: 0 - NOT SPECIFIED 1 - RAPID 2 - DELAYED   SEVERITY: 1 - CONTRAINDICATED 2 - MAJOR 3 - MODERATE

phenelzine	1	1	1	May result in hypertensive crisis (headache, hyperpyrexia, hypertension).
procarbazine	1	1	2	May result in hypertensive crisis (headache, hyperpyrexia, hypertension).
selegiline	1	1	1	May result in hypertensive crisis (headache, hyperpyrexia, hypertension) and serotonin syndrome (hypertension, hyperthermia, myoclonus, mental status changes).
toloxatone	1	1	2	May result in hypertensive crisis (headache, hyperpyrexia, hypertension).
tranylcypromine	1	1	1	May result in hypertensive crisis (headache, hyperpyrexia, hypertension).
ARIPIPRAZOLE				
carbamazepine	2	3	2	May result in decreased aripiprazole concentrations.
ketoconazole	2	3	2	May result in increased aripiprazole concentrations.
quinidine	2	3	2	May result in increased aripiprazole levels.
ASPIRIN				
anisindione	2	2	1	May result in increased risk of bleeding.
betamethasone	2	3	2	May result in increased risk of gastrointestinal ulceration and subtherapeutic aspirin serum concentrations.
captopril	1	3	1	May result in decreased captopril effectiveness.
celecoxib	2	3	2	May result in increased risk of gastrointestinal bleeding.

chlorpropamide	2	3	2	May result in hypoglycemia (CNS depression, seizures).
cortisone	2	3	2	May result in increased risk of gastrointestinal ulceration and subtherapeutic aspirin serum concentrations.
deflazacort	2	3	2	May result in increased risk of gastrointestinal ulceration and subtherapeutic aspirin serum concentrations.
delapril	1	3	1	May result in decreased delapril effectiveness.
desvenlafaxine	0	2	2	May result in increased risk of bleeding.
dexamethasone	2	3	2	May result in increased risk of gastrointestinal ulceration and subtherapeutic aspirin serum concentrations.
dicumarol	2	2	2	May result in increased risk of bleeding.
diltiazem	2	3	2	May result in prolongation of bleeding time.
enalapril maleate	1	3	1	May result in decreased effectiveness of enalapril.
enalaprilat	1	3	1	May result in decreased effectiveness of enalapril.
eptifibatide	1	2	2	May result in increased risk of bleeding.
ethanol	1	3	2	May result in increased gastrointestinal blood loss.
furosemide	1	3	2	May result in blunting of the diuretic effect of furosemide.
ginkgo	0	2	2	May result in increased risk of bleeding.
glyburide	2	3	2	May result in increased risk for hypoglycemia.
heparin	1	2	1	May result in increased risk of bleeding.

ibuprofen	1	3	2	May result in decreased antiplatelet effect of aspirin.
imidapril	1	3	1	May result in decreased imidapril effectiveness.
lisinopril	1	3	2	May result in decreased lisinopril effectiveness.
LMWHs (ardeparin, certoparin, dalteparin, danaparoid, enoxaparin, nadroparin, parnaparin, reviparin, tinzaparin)	1	3	2	May result in increased risk of bleeding and an increased risk of hematoma when neuraxial anesthesia is employed.
methotrexate	1	2	2	May result in methotrexate toxicity (leukopenia, thrombocytopenia, anemia, nephrotoxicity, mucosal ulcerations).
methylprednisolone	2	3	2	May result in increased risk of gastrointestinal ulceration and subtherapeutic aspirin serum concentrations.
nitroglycerin	1	3	2	May result in increased nitroglycerin concentrations and additive platelet function depression.
paramethasone	2	3	2	May result in increased risk of gastrointestinal ulceration and subtherapeutic aspirin serum concentrations.
phenprocoumon	2	2	1	May result in increased risk of bleeding.
prednisolone	2	3	2	May result in increased risk of gastrointestinal ulceration and subtherapeutic aspirin serum concentrations.
prednisone	2	3	2	May result in increased risk of gastrointestinal ulceration and subtherapeutic aspirin serum concentrations.
probenecid	2	3	2	May result in reversal of the uricosuric effects of the other drug.

rofecoxib	2	3	2	May result in increased risk of gastrointestinal bleeding.
SSRIs (*citalopram, clovoxamin, femoxetine, flexinoxan, fluoxetine, fluvoxamine, nefazodone, paroxetine, sertraline, venlafaxine, zimeldine*)	0	3	2	May result in increased risk of bleeding.
streptokinase	2	3	1	May result in increased risk of hemorrhagic complications.
tamarind	1	3	2	May result in increased salicylate toxicity.
temocapril	1	3	1	May result in decreased temocapril effectiveness.
tenecteplase	1	3	2	May result in increased risk of bleeding.
ticlopidine	2	2	2	May result in increased risk of bleeding.
tirofiban	1	3	2	May result in increased risk of bleeding.
tolbutamide	2	3	2	May result in hypoglycemia (CNS depression, seizures).
triamcinolone	2	3	2	May result in increased risk of gastrointestinal ulceration and subtherapeutic aspirin serum concentrations.
valproic acid	2	3	2	May result in increased free valproic acid concentrations.
varicella virus vaccine	2	2	2	May result in enhanced risk of developing Reye's syndrome.
verapamil	2	3	2	May result in increased risk of bleeding.

ONSET: 0 - NOT SPECIFIED 1 - RAPID 2 - DELAYED   SEVERITY: 1 - CONTRAINDICATED 2 - MAJOR 3 - MODERATE

warfarin	2	2	1	May result in increased risk of bleeding.
zimeldine	0	3	2	May result in increased risk of bleeding.

ATENOLOL

α-1 Blockers (*alfuzosin, bunazosin, doxazosin, moxisylate, phenoxybenzamine, phentolamine, prazosin, tamsulosin, terazosin, trimazosin, urapidil*)	1	3	2	May result in exaggerated hypotensive response to the first dose of the α-blocker.
Antidiabetic Agents (*acarbose, acetohexamide, benfluorex, chlorpropamide, glicazide, glimepiride, glipizide, gliquidone, glyburide, guar gum, insulin, insulin aspart, recombinant, insulin glulisine, insulin lispro, recombinant, metformin, miglitol, repaglinide, tolazamide, tolbutamide, troglitazone*)	2	3	2	May result in hypoglycemia, hyperglycemia, or hypertension.
arbutamine	1	3	2	May result in attenuation of the response to arbutamine by the β-blocker, resulting in unreliable arbutamine test results.
CCBs, Dihydropyridine (*amlodipine, felodipine, lacidipine, lercanidipine, manidipine, nicardipine, nifedipine, nilvadipine, nimodipine, nisoldipine, nitrendipine, pranidipine*)	1	3	2	May result in hypotension and/or bradycardia.

clonidine	2	2	2	May result in exaggerated clonidine withdrawal response (acute hypertension).
digoxin	2	3	2	May result in AV block and possible digoxin toxicity.
diltiazem	1	3	2	May result in increased risk of hypotension, bradycardia, AV conduction disturbances.
disopyramide	1	3	2	May result in bradycardia, decreased cardiac output.
fentanyl	1	2	2	May result in severe hypotension.
mibefradil	2	3	2	May result in hypotension, bradycardia, and AV conduction disturbances.
quinidine	1	3	2	May result in bradycardia, hypotension.
St. John's wort	2	3	2	May result in decreased effectiveness of β-blockers.
verapamil	1	2	2	May result in hypotension, bradycardia.
ATOMOXETINE				
albuterol	0	2	2	May result in increased heart rate and blood pressure.
amitriptyline	0	3	2	May result in increased atomoxetine steady-state plasma concentrations.
amoxapine	0	3	2	May result in increased atomoxetine steady-state plasma concentrations.
clomipramine	0	3	2	May result in increased atomoxetine steady-state plasma concentrations.

desipramine	0	3	2	May result in increased atomoxetine steady-state plasma concentrations.
dibenzepin	0	3	2	May result in increased atomoxetine steady-state plasma concentrations.
dothiepin	0	3	2	May result in increased atomoxetine steady-state plasma concentrations.
doxepin	0	3	2	May result in increased atomoxetine steady-state plasma concentrations.
imipramine	0	3	2	May result in increased atomoxetine steady-state plasma concentrations.
lofepramine	0	3	2	May result in increased atomoxetine steady-state plasma concentrations.
nortriptyline	0	3	2	May result in increased atomoxetine steady-state plasma concentrations.
opipramol	0	3	2	May result in increased atomoxetine steady-state plasma concentrations.
protriptyline	0	3	2	May result in increased atomoxetine steady-state plasma concentrations.
tianeptine	0	3	2	May result in increased atomoxetine steady-state plasma concentrations.
trimipramine	0	3	2	May result in increased atomoxetine steady-state plasma concentrations.

ATORVASTATIN

Drug	Onset	Severity	Documentation	Description
aliskiren	2	3	2	May result in increased aliskiren exposure and plasma concentrations.
amprenavir	2	3	2	May result in increased risk of myopathy or rhabdomyolysis.
bezafibrate	2	2	2	May result in increased risk of myopathy or rhabdomyolysis.
bosentan	1	3	2	May result in reduced plasma concentrations and reduced efficacy of atorvastatin.
ciprofibrate	2	2	2	May result in increased risk of myopathy or rhabdomyolysis.
clarithromycin	2	2	2	May result in increased atorvastatin exposure and an increased risk of myopathy or rhabdomyolysis.
clofibrate	2	2	2	May result in increased risk of myopathy or rhabdomyolysis.
cyclosporine	2	2	2	May result in increased risk of myopathy or rhabdomyolysis.
dalfopristin	2	2	2	May result in increased risk of myopathy or rhabdomyolysis.

ONSET: 0 - NOT SPECIFIED, 1 - RAPID, 2 - DELAYED   SEVERITY: 1 - CONTRAINDICATED, 2 - MAJOR, 3 - MODERATE

darunavir	0	3	1	May result in increased atorvastatin plasma concentrations.
digoxin	2	3	2	May result in increased plasma concentrations of digoxin.
diltiazem	2	2	2	May result in increased risk of rhabdomyolysis.
efavirenz	2	3	1	May result in decreased atorvastatin plasma concentrations.
erythromycin	2	2	2	May result in increased atorvastatin exposure and an increased risk of myopathy or rhabdomyolysis.
fenofibrate	0	2	2	May result in increased risk of myopathy or rhabdomyolysis.
fosamprenavir	2	2	2	May result in increased risk of myopathy or rhabdomyolysis.
fosphenytoin	2	3	2	May result in loss of atorvastatin efficacy.
fusidic acid	2	2	2	May result in increased plasma concentrations of fusidic acid and atorvastatin.
gemfibrozil	2	2	1	May result in increased atorvastatin levels and an increased risk of myopathy or rhabdomyolysis.
grapefruit juice	1	3	2	May result in increased bioavailability of atorvastatin resulting in an increased risk of myopathy or rhabdomyolysis.
indinavir	2	2	2	May result in increased risk of myopathy or rhabdomyolysis.
itraconazole	2	2	2	May result in increased risk of myopathy or rhabdomyolysis.

lopinavir	2	2	1	May result in increased exposure to atorvastatin with increased risk of side effects.
mibefradil	2	2	2	May result in increased risk of myopathy and/or rhabdomyolysis.
nefazodone	2	2	2	May result in increased risk of myopathy or rhabdomyolysis.
nelfinavir	2	2	2	May result in increased risk of myopathy or rhabdomyolysis.
oat bran	2	3	2	May result in reduced effectiveness of HMG CoA reductase inhibitors.
pectin	2	3	2	May result in reduced effectiveness of HMG CoA reductase inhibitors.
phenytoin	2	3	2	May result in loss of atorvastatin efficacy.
pioglitazone	2	3	2	May result in reduced pioglitazone bioavailability and increased risk of hyperglycemia.
quinupristin	2	2	2	May result in increased risk of myopathy or rhabdomyolysis.
rifampin	1	3	2	May result in decreased atorvastatin concentration.
ritonavir	2	3	2	May result in increased risk of myopathy or rhabdomyolysis.

ONSET: 0 - NOT SPECIFIED 1 - RAPID 2 - DELAYED   SEVERITY: 1 - CONTRAINDICATED 2 - MAJOR 3 - MODERATE

saquinavir	2	2	2	May result in increased risk of myopathy or rhabdomyolysis.
St. John's wort	2	3	2	May result in reduced effectiveness of atorvastatin.
telithromycin	2	2	2	May result in increased atorvastatin plasma levels.
tipranavir	2	2	1	May result in increased exposure to atorvastatin with increased risk of side effects.
voriconazole	0	3	2	May result in increased plasma concentrations of atorvastatin.

AZELASTINE

| cimetidine | 2 | 3 | 2 | May result in increased risk of azelastine adverse effects (increased somnolence, headache, bitter taste). |

AZITHROMYCIN

amiodarone	2	2	2	May result in increased risk of cardiotoxicity (QT prolongation, torsades de pointes, cardiac arrest).
digoxin	2	3	2	May result in digoxin toxicity (vomiting, cardiac arrhythmias).
disopyramide	2	2	2	May result in cardiac arrhythmias (prolonged QTc, ventricular tachycardia).
Ergot Derivatives (dihydroergotamine, ergoloid mesylates, ergonovine, ergotamine, methylergonovine, methysergide)	2	1	2	May result in increased risk of acute ergotism (nausea, vomiting, vasospastic ischemia).

Drug	Onset	Severity		Effect
fentanyl	2	3	2	May result in increased or prolonged opioid effects (CNS depression, respiratory depression).
nelfinavir	2	3	2	May result in increased azithromycin plasma concentrations and risk of adverse effects (diarrhea, ototoxicity, hepatotoxicity).
rifabutin	2	3	2	May result in increased risk of rifabutin toxicity (rash, GI disturbances, hematologic abnormalities).
theophylline	2	3	2	May result in increased serum theophylline concentrations.
warfarin	2	3	2	May result in increased risk of bleeding.
BENAZEPRIL				
aliskiren	0	3	2	May result in hyperkalemia.
amiloride	2	2	2	May result in hyperkalemia.
bupivacaine	2	3	2	May result in bradycardia and hypotension with loss of consciousness.
capsaicin	1	3	2	May result in increased risk of cough.
lithium	2	3	2	May result in lithium toxicity (weakness, tremor, excessive thirst, confusion) and/or nephrotoxicity.
Loop Diuretics (azosemide, bumetanide, ethacrynic acid, furosemide, piretanide, torsemide)	1	3	2	May result in postural hypotension (first dose).
nesiritide	2	3	2	May result in increased symptomatic hypotension.

ONSET: 0 – NOT SPECIFIED 1 – RAPID 2 – DELAYED   SEVERITY: 1 – CONTRAINDICATED 2 – MAJOR 3 – MODERATE

Drug			Effect
NSAIDs (aceclofenac, acemetacin, alclofenac, apazone, aspirin, benoxaprofen, bromfenac, bufexamac, carprofen, celecoxib, clometacin, clonixin, dexketoprofen, diclofenac, diflunisal, dipyrone, dofetilide, droxicam, etodolac, etofenamate, felbinac, fenbufen, fenoprofen, fentiazac, floctafenine, flufenamic acid, flurbiprofen, ibuprofen, indomethacin, indoprofen, isoxicam, ketoprofen, ketorolac, lornoxicam, meclofenamate, mefanamic acid, meloxicam, nabumetone, naproxen, niflumic acid, nimesulide, oxaprozin, oxyphenbutazone, phenylbutazone, pirazolac, piroxicam, pirprofen, propyphenazon, proquazone, rofecoxib, sulindac, suprofen, tenidap, tenoxicam, tiaprofenic acid, ticrynafen, tolmetin, zomepirac)	2	3	2	May result in decreased antihypertensive and natriuretic effects.
potassium	2	2	2	May result in hyperkalemia.
Thiazide Diuretics (bemetizide, bendroflumethiazide, benzthiazide, buthiazide, chlorthiazide, chlorthalidone, clopamide, cyclopenthiazide,	1	3	2	May result in postural hypotension (first dose).

cyclothiazide, HCTZ, hydroflumethiazide, indapamide, methyclothiazide, metolazone, polythiazide, quinethazone, trichlormethiazide, xipamide)				
BETAMETHASONE				
alcuronium	2	3	2	May result in decreased alcuronium effectiveness; prolonged muscle weakness and myopathy.
aspirin	2	3	2	May result in increased risk of gastrointestinal ulceration and subtherapeutic aspirin serum concentrations.
atracurium	2	3	2	May result in decreased atracurium effectiveness; prolonged muscle weakness and myopathy.
Contraceptives, Combination (ethinyl estradiol, etonogestrel, mestranol, norelgestromin, norethindrone, norgestrel)	2	3	2	May result in increased corticosteroid effects.
FLQs (alatrofloxacin, balofloxacin, cinoxacin, ciprofloxacin, clinafloxacin, enoxacin, fleroxacin, flumequine, gemifloxacin, grepafloxacin, levofloxacin, lomefloxacin, moxifloxacin, norfloxacin, ofloxacin, pefloxacin, prulifloxacin, rosoxacin, rufloxacin, sparfloxacin, temafloxacin, tosufloxacin, trovafloxacin)	2	3	1	May result in increased risk for tendon rupture.

fosphenytoin	2	3	2	May result in decreased betamethasone effectiveness.
gallamine	2	3	2	May result in decreased gallamine effectiveness; prolonged muscle weakness and myopathy.
hexafluorenium	2	3	2	May result in decreased hexafluorenium bromide effectiveness; prolonged muscle weakness and myopathy.
itraconazole	2	3	2	May result in increased corticosteroid plasma concentrations and increased risk of corticosteroid side effects (myopathy, glucose intolerance, Cushing's syndrome).
licorice	2	3	2	May result in increased risk of corticosteroid adverse effects.
metocurine	2	3	2	May result in decreased metocurine effectiveness; prolonged muscle weakness and myopathy.
phenobarbital	2	3	2	May result in decreased betamethasone effectiveness.
phenytoin	2	3	2	May result in decreased betamethasone effectiveness.
primidone	2	3	2	May result in decreased betamethasone effectiveness.
quetiapine	0	2	2	May result in decreased serum quetiapine concentrations.
rifampin	2	3	2	May result in decreased betamethasone effectiveness.
rifapentine	2	3	2	May result in decreased corticosteroid effectiveness.
rotavirus vaccine, live	2	1	1	May result in increased risk of infection by the live vaccine.

saiboku-to	2	3	2	May result in enhanced and prolonged effect of corticosteroids.

BISOPROLOL

α-1 Blockers (*alfuzosin, bunazosin, doxazosin, moxisylate, phenoxybenzamine, phentolamine, prazosin, tamsulosin, terazosin, trimazosin, urapidil*)	1	3	2	May result in exaggerated hypotensive response to the first dose of the α-blocker.
Antidiabetic Agents (*acarbose, acetohexamide, benfluorex, chlorpropamide, glicazide, glimepiride, glipizide, gliquidone, glyburide, guar gum, insulin, insulin aspart, recombinant, insulin glulisine, insulin lispro, recombinant, metformin, miglitol, repaglinide, tolazamide, tolbutamide, troglitazone*)	2	3	2	May result in hypoglycemia, hyperglycemia, or hypertension.
arbutamine	1	3	2	May result in attenuation of the response to arbutamine by the β-blocker, resulting in unreliable arbutamine test results.
CCBs, Dihydropyridine (*amlodipine, felodipine, lacidipine, lercanidipine, manidipine, nicardipine, nifedipine, nilvadipine, nimodipine, nisoldipine, nitrendipine, prandipine*)	1	3	2	May result in hypotension and/or bradycardia.

ONSET: 0 - NOT SPECIFIED 1 - RAPID 2 - DELAYED   SEVERITY: 1 - CONTRAINDICATED 2 - MAJOR 3 - MODERATE

digoxin	2	3	2	May result in AV block and possible digoxin toxicity.
diltiazem	1	3	2	May result in increased risk of hypotension, bradycardia, AV conduction disturbances.
fentanyl	1	2	2	May result in severe hypotension.
methyldopa	1	3	2	May result in exaggerated hypertensive response, tachycardia, or arrhythmias during physiologic stress or exposure to exogenous catecholamines.
mibefradil	2	3	2	May result in hypotension, bradycardia, and AV conduction disturbances.
rifapentine	2	3	2	May result in decreased β-blocker effectiveness.
St. John's wort	2	3	2	May result in decreased β-blocker effectiveness.
verapamil	1	2	2	May result in hypotension, bradycardia.
BUDESONIDE				
erythromycin	0	3	2	May result in increased budesonide plasma concentrations.
grapefruit juice	0	3	1	May result in two-fold increased systemic exposure of budesonide possibly increased cortisol suppression.
itraconazole	0	3	2	May result in increased budesonide plasma concentrations.
ketoconazole	1	3	2	May result in increased budesonide plasma concentrations.

BUPRENORPHINE

alfentanil	2	2	2	May result in precipitation of withdrawal symptoms (abdominal cramps, nausea, vomiting, lacrimation, rhinorrhea, anxiety, restlessness, elevation of temperature or piloerection).
alphaprodine	2	2	2	May result in precipitation of withdrawal symptoms (abdominal cramps, nausea, vomiting, lacrimation, rhinorrhea, anxiety, restlessness, elevation of temperature or piloerection).
codeine	2	2	2	May result in precipitation of withdrawal symptoms (abdominal cramps, nausea, vomiting, lacrimation, rhinorrhea, anxiety, restlessness, elevation of temperature or piloerection).
diazepam	1	2	2	May result in respiratory and cardiovascular collapse.
dihydrocodeine	2	2	2	May result in precipitation of withdrawal symptoms (abdominal cramps, nausea, vomiting, lacrimation, rhinorrhea, anxiety, restlessness, elevation of temperature or piloerection).
fentanyl	2	2	2	May result in precipitation of withdrawal symptoms (abdominal cramps, nausea, vomiting, lacrimation, rhinorrhea, anxiety, restlessness, elevation of temperature or piloerection).

ONSET: 0 = NOT SPECIFIED 1 = RAPID 2 = DELAYED   SEVERITY: 1 = CONTRAINDICATED 2 = MAJOR 3 = MODERATE

hydrocodone	2	2	2	May result in precipitation of withdrawal symptoms (abdominal cramps, nausea, vomiting, lacrimation, rhinorrhea, anxiety, restlessness, elevation of temperature or piloerection).
hydromorphone	2	2	2	May result in precipitation of withdrawal symptoms (abdominal cramps, nausea, vomiting, lacrimation, rhinorrhea, anxiety, restlessness, elevation of temperature or piloerection).
levorphanol	2	2	2	May result in precipitation of withdrawal symptoms (abdominal cramps, nausea, vomiting, lacrimation, rhinorrhea, anxiety, restlessness, elevation of temperature or piloerection).
meperidine	2	2	2	May result in precipitation of withdrawal symptoms (abdominal cramps, nausea, vomiting, lacrimation, rhinorrhea, anxiety, restlessness, elevation of temperature or piloerection).
methadone	2	2	2	May result in precipitation of withdrawal symptoms (abdominal cramps, nausea, vomiting, lacrimation, rhinorrhea, anxiety, restlessness, elevation of temperature or piloerection).
morphine	2	2	2	May result in precipitation of withdrawal symptoms (abdominal cramps, nausea, vomiting, lacrimation, rhinorrhea, anxiety, restlessness, elevation of temperature or piloerection).

morphine sulfate liposome	2	2	2	May result in precipitation of withdrawal symptoms (abdominal cramps, nausea, vomiting, lacrimation, rhinorrhea, anxiety, restlessness, elevation of temperature or piloerection).
oxycodone	2	2	2	May result in precipitation of withdrawal symptoms (abdominal cramps, nausea, vomiting, lacrimation, rhinorrhea, anxiety, restlessness, elevation of temperature or piloerection).
oxymorphone	2	2	2	May result in precipitation of withdrawal symptoms (abdominal cramps, nausea, vomiting, lacrimation, rhinorrhea, anxiety, restlessness, elevation of temperature or piloerection).
propoxyphene	2	2	2	May result in precipitation of withdrawal symptoms (abdominal cramps, nausea, vomiting, lacrimation, rhinorrhea, anxiety, restlessness, elevation of temperature or piloerection).
sufentanil	2	2	2	May result in precipitation of withdrawal symptoms (abdominal cramps, nausea, vomiting, lacrimation, rhinorrhea, anxiety, restlessness, elevation of temperature or piloerection).
BUPROPION				
amantadine	2	3	2	May result in increased risk of adverse effects (nausea, vomiting, excitation, restlessness, postural hypotension).

ONSET: 0 – NOT SPECIFIED 1 – RAPID 2 – DELAYED   SEVERITY: 1 – CONTRAINDICATED 2 – MAJOR 3 – MODERATE

carbimazole	2	2	2	May result in increased risk of hepatotoxicity.
desipramine	2	3	2	May result in increased plasma levels of desipramine.
ethanol	2	2	2	May result in increased risk of seizures.
flecainide	2	3	2	May result in increased plasma levels of flecainide.
fluoxetine	2	3	2	May result in increased plasma levels of fluoxetine.
guanfacine	2	3	2	May result in increased risk of seizure activity in presence of no previous history of seizures.
haloperidol	2	3	2	May result in increased plasma levels of haloperidol.
iproniazid	1	1	2	May result in bupropion toxicity (seizures, agitation, psychotic changes).
levodopa	2	3	1	May result in increased risk of adverse effects (nausea, vomiting, excitation, restlessness, postural tremor).
linezolid	0	2	2	May result in increased risk of serotonin syndrome (hyperthermia, hyperreflexia, myoclonus, mental status changes).
lopinavir	2	3	1	May result in decreased bupropion plasma concentrations.
metoprolol	2	3	2	May result in increased plasma levels of metoprolol.
nialamide	1	1	2	May result in bupropion toxicity (seizures, agitation, psychotic changes).
nortriptyline	2	3	2	May result in increased plasma levels of nortriptyline.

pargyline	1	1	2	May result in bupropion toxicity (seizures, agitation, psychotic changes).
paroxetine	2	3	2	May result in increased plasma levels of paroxetine.
procarbazine	1	1	2	May result in bupropion toxicity (seizures, agitation, psychotic changes).
propafenone	2	3	2	May result in increased plasma levels of propafenone.
risperidone	2	3	2	May result in increased plasma levels of risperidone.
sertraline	2	3	2	May result in increased plasma levels of sertraline.
theophylline	0	2	2	May result in increased plasma concentrations of theophylline.
thioridazine	2	3	2	May result in increased plasma levels of thioridazine.
toloxatone	1	1	2	May result in bupropion toxicity (seizures, agitation, psychotic changes).
zolpidem	2	3	2	May result in increased risk of hallucinations.
BUSPIRONE				
clozapine	2	2	2	May result in increased risk of gastrointestinal bleeding and hyperglycemia.
diltiazem	1	3	2	May result in increased risk of enhanced buspirone effects.

ONSET: 0 - NOT SPECIFIED, 1 - RAPID, 2 - DELAYED   SEVERITY: 1 - CONTRAINDICATED, 2 - MAJOR, 3 - MODERATE

erythromycin	1	3	2	May result in increased buspirone plasma concentrations; increased buspirone side effects (impaired psychomotor performance, sedation).
fluoxetine	2	3	2	May result in worsening of psychiatric symptoms.
ginkgo	2	3	2	May result in changes in mental status.
grapefruit juice	1	3	2	May result in increased risk of buspirone toxicity (dizziness, sedation).
iproniazid	1	2	2	May result in hypertensive crisis.
itraconazole	1	3	2	May result in increased buspirone plasma concentrations; increased buspirone side effects (impaired psychomotor performance, sedation).
nefazodone	1	3	2	May result in increased buspirone plasma concentrations.
nialamide	1	2	2	May result in hypertensive crisis.
pargyline	1	2	2	May result in hypertensive crisis.
phenelzine	1	1	2	May result in hypertensive crisis.
procarbazine	1	2	2	May result in hypertensive crisis.
rifampin	1	3	2	May result in reduced anxiolytic effects of buspirone.
selegiline	1	2	2	May result in hypertensive crisis.
St. John's wort	2	3	2	May result in increased risk of serotonin syndrome (hypertension, hyperthermia, myoclonus, mental status changes) or hypomania.

toloxatone	1	2	2	May result in hypertensive crisis.
tranylcypromine	1	1	2	May result in hypertensive crisis.
verapamil	1	3	2	May result in increased risk of enhanced buspirone effects.

BUTALBITAL

BZDs (*adinazolam, alprazolam, bromazepam, brotizolam, chlordiazepoxide, clobazam, clonazepam, clorazepate, diazepam, estazolam, flunitrazepam, flurazepam, halazepam, ketazolam, lorazepam, lormetazepam, lormetazepam, medazepam, midazolam, nitrazepam, nordazepam, oxazepam, prazepam, temazepam, triazolam*)	0	2	2	May result in additive respiratory depression.
cannabis	1	3	2	May result in increased CNS depression.
dicumarol	2	2	2	May result in decreased anticoagulant effectiveness.
ethanol	1	3	2	May result in excessive CNS depression.
imipramine	2	3	2	May result in decreased efficacy of imipramine.

Opioid Analgesics (*alfentanil, anileridine, codeine, fentanyl, hydrocodone, hydromorphone, levorphanol, meperidine, morphine, morphine sulfate liposome, oxycodone, oxymorphone, propoxyphene, remifentanil, sufentanil*)	0	2	2	May result in additive respiratory depression.
phenprocoumon	2	2	2	May result in decreased anticoagulant effectiveness.
prednisone	2	3	2	May result in decreased therapeutic effect of prednisone.
quetiapine	0	2	2	May result in decreased serum quetiapine concentrations.
warfarin	2	3	2	May result in decreased anticoagulant effectiveness.
CAFFEINE				
ciprofloxacin	2	3	2	May result in increased caffeine concentrations and enhanced CNS stimulation.
clozapine	2	3	2	May result in increased risk of clozapine toxicity (sedation, seizures, hypotension).
Contraceptives, Combination (*ethinyl estradiol, etonogestrel, mestranol, norelgestromin, norethindrone, norgestrel*)	1	3	2	May result in enhanced CNS stimulation.
enoxacin	2	3	2	May result in increased caffeine concentrations and enhanced CNS stimulation.

grepafloxacin	2	3	2	May result in increased caffeine concentrations and enhanced CNS stimulation.
theophylline	2	3	2	May result in increased theophylline concentrations and toxicity (nausea, vomiting, palpitations, seizures).

CARISOPRODOL

Opioid Analgesics (*alfentanil, anileridine, codeine, fentanyl, hydrocodone, hydromorphone, levorphanol, meperidine, morphine, morphine sulfate liposome, oxycodone, oxymorphone, propoxyphene, remifentanil, sufentanil*)	0	2	2	May result in additive respiratory depression.

CARVEDILOL

α-1 Blockers (*alfuzosin, bunazosin, doxazosin, moxisylate, phenoxybenzamine, phentolamine, prazosin, tamsulosin, terazosin, trimazosin, urapidil*)	1	3	2	May result in exaggerated hypotensive response to the first dose of the α-blocker.

INTERACTING DRUG	ONSET	SEVERITY	EVIDENCE	WARNING
Antidiabetic Agents (*acarbose, acetohexamide, benfluorex, chlorpropamide, glicazide, glimepiride, glipizide, gliquidone, glyburide, guar gum, insulin, insulin aspart, recombinant, insulin glulisine, insulin lispro, recombinant, metformin, miglitol, repaglinide, tolazamide, tolbutamide, troglitazone*)	2	3	2	May result in hypoglycemia, hyperglycemia, or hypertension.
arbutamine	1	3	2	May result in attenuation of the response to arbutamine by the β-blocker, resulting in unreliable arbutamine test results.
CCBs, Dihydropyridine (*amlodipine, felodipine, lacidipine, lercanidipine, manidipine, nicardipine, nifedipine, nilvadipine, nimodipine, nisoldipine, nitrendipine, prandipine*)	1	3	2	May result in hypotension and/or bradycardia.
cimetidine	1	3	2	May result in increased adverse effects of carvedilol (dizziness, insomnia, GI symptoms, postural hypotension).
digoxin	2	3	2	May result in AV block and possible digoxin toxicity.
diltiazem	1	3	2	May result in increased risk of hypotension, bradycardia, AV conduction disturbances.
epinephrine	1	2	2	May result in hypertension, bradycardia, resistance to epinephrine in anaphylaxis.

	Onset	Severity		Description
fentanyl	1	2	2	May result in severe hypotension.
mibefradil	2	3	2	May result in hypotension, bradycardia, and AV conduction disturbances.
rifampin	1	3	2	May result in decreased therapeutic response to carvedilol.
rifapentine	2	3	2	May result in decreased effectiveness of β-blockers.
St. John's wort	2	3	2	May result in decreased effectiveness of β-blockers.
verapamil	1	2	2	May result in hypotension, bradycardia.

CEFUROXIME

none reported

CELECOXIB

ACE Inhibitors (alacepril, benazepril, captopril, cilazapril, delapril, enalapril maleate, enalaprilat, fosinopril, imidapril, lisinopril, moexipril, pentopril, perindopril, quinapril, ramipril, spirapril, temocapril, trandolapril, zofenopril)	2	3	2	May result in decreased antihypertensive and natriuretic effects.
aspirin	2	3	2	May result in increased risk of gastrointestinal bleeding.
desvenlafaxine	0	2	2	May result in increased risk of bleeding.
diltiazem	2	3	2	May result in loss of blood pressure control.

ONSET: 0 = NOT SPECIFIED, 1 = RAPID, 2 = DELAYED   SEVERITY: 1 = CONTRAINDICATED, 2 = MAJOR, 3 = MODERATE

fluconazole	2	3	2	May result in increased celecoxib plasma concentrations.
lithium	2	3	2	May result in increased lithium plasma concentrations and an increased risk of lithium toxicity (weakness, tremor, excessive thirst, confusion).
Loop Diuretics (*azosemide, bumetanide, ethacrynic acid, furosemide, piretanide, torsemide*)	2	3	2	May result in decreased diuretic and antihypertensive efficacy.
SSRIs (*citalopram, clovoxamine, femoxetine, fleinoxan, fluoxetine, nefazodone, paroxetine, sertraline, venlafaxine, zimeldine*)	0	3	2	May result in increased risk of bleeding.
Thiazide Diuretics (*bemetizide, bendroflumethiazide, benzthiazide, buthiazide, chlorthiazide, chlorthalidone, clopamide, cyclopenthiazide, cyclothiazide, HCTZ, hydroflumethiazide, indapamide, methyclothiazide, metolazone, polythiazide, quinethazone, trichlormethiazide, xipamide*)	2	3	2	May result in decreased diuretic and antihypertensive efficacy.
venlafaxine	0	3	2	May result in increased risk of bleeding.
warfarin	2	2	2	May result in increased risk of bleeding.

CEPHALEXIN

cholestyramine	1	3	2	May result in decreased cephalexin effectiveness.
metformin	0	3	2	May result in increased metformin plasma levels and may increase risk of metformin side effects (nausea, vomiting, diarrhea, asthenia, headache).

CHLORTHALIDONE

ACE Inhibitors (*alacepril, benazepril, captopril, cilazapril, delapril, enalapril maleate, enalaprilat, fosinopril, imidapril, lisinopril, moexipril, pentopril, perindopril, quinapril, ramipril, spirapril, temocapril, trandolapril, zofenopril*)	1	3	2	May result in postural hypotension (first dose).
calcitriol	2	3	2	May result in hypercalcemia.
chlorpropamide	2	3	1	May result in decreased chlorpropamide effectiveness.
Digitalis Glycosides (*acetydigoxin, deslanoside, digitalis, digitoxin, digoxin, metildigoxin*)	2	2	1	May result in digitalis toxicity (nausea, vomiting, arrhythmias).
gossypol	2	3	2	May result in increased risk of hypokalemia.
licorice	2	3	2	May result in increased risk of hypokalemia and/or reduced effectiveness of the diuretic.

ONSET: 0 - NOT SPECIFIED 1 - RAPID 2 - DELAYED   SEVERITY: 1 - CONTRAINDICATED 2 - MAJOR 3 - MODERATE

NSAIDs (aceclofenac, acemetacin, alclofenac, apazone, benoxaprofen, bromfenac, bufexamac, carprofen, celecoxib, clometacin, clonixin, dexketoprofen, diclofenac, diflunisal, dipyrone, dofetilide, droxicam, etodolac, etofenamate, felbinac, fenbufen, fenoprofen, fentiazac, floctafenine, flufenamic acid, flurbiprofen, ibuprofen, indomethacin, indoprofen, isoxicam, ketoprofen, ketorolac, lornoxicam, meclofenamate, mefanamic acid, meloxicam, nabumetone, naproxen, niflumic acid, nimesulide, oxaprozin, oxyphenbutazone, phenylbutazone, pirazolac, piroxicam, pirprofen, propyphenazon, proquazone, rofecoxib, sulindac, suprofen, tenidap, tenoxicam, tiaprofenic acid, ticrynafen, tolmetin, zomepirac)	2	3	2	May result in decreased diuretic and antihypertensive efficacy.
sotalol	0	2	2	May result in increased risk of cardiotoxicity (QT prolongation, torsades de pointes, cardiac arrest).

CIPROFLOXACIN

Drug	Onset	Severity		Effect
Antacids (*aluminum carbonate, basic, aluminum hydroxide, aluminum phosphate, dihydroxyaluminum aminoacetate, dihydroxyaluminum sodium carbonate, fludrocortisone, fluocortolone, hydrocortisone, magaldrate, magnesium carbonate, magnesium hydroxide, magnesium oxide, magnesium trisilicate*)	1	3	2	May result in decreased ciprofloxacin effectiveness.
Antidiabetic Agents (*acarbose, acetohexamide, benfluorex, chlorpropamide, glicazide, glimepiride, glipizide, gliquidone, glyburide, guar gum, insulin, insulin aspart, recombinant, insulin glulisine, insulin lispro, recombinant, metformin, miglitol, repaglinide, tolazamide, tolbutamide, troglitazone*)	1	2	1	May result in changes in blood glucose and increased risk of hypoglycemia or hyperglycemia.
caffeine	2	3	2	May result in increased caffeine concentrations and enhanced CNS stimulation.
calcium	1	3	2	May result in decreased ciprofloxacin efficacy.

ONSET: 0 – NOT SPECIFIED 1 – RAPID 2 – DELAYED   SEVERITY: 1 – CONTRAINDICATED 2 – MAJOR 3 – MODERATE

Corticosteroids (*betamethasone, corticotropin, cortisone, cosyntropin, deflazacort, dexamethasone, methylprednisolone, paramethasone, prednisolone, prednisone, triamcinolone*)	2	3	1	May result in increased risk for tendon rupture.
cyclosporine	2	3	1	May result in increased cyclosporine blood levels, loss of cyclosporine therapeutic effect or transient elevations in serum creatinine.
dairy food	1	3	2	May result in decreased ciprofloxacin concentrations.
didanosine	1	3	2	May result in loss of ciprofloxacin efficacy.
dutasteride	0	3	2	May result in increased dutasteride plasma concentrations.
fosphenytoin	2	3	2	May result in increased or decreased phenytoin levels.
indomethacin	1	2	2	May result in formation of indomethacin-ciprofloxacin precipitate deposits in the eye.
olanzapine	2	3	2	May result in increased risk of olanzapine toxicity (increased sedation, orthostatic hypotension).
phenytoin	2	3	2	May result in increased or decreased phenytoin levels.
rasagiline	0	3	1	May result in increased rasagiline exposure and risk of rasagiline adverse effects.
rifapentine	2	3	2	May result in decreased ciprofloxacin effectiveness.
ropinirole	2	3	1	May result in increased risk of ropinirole adverse effects (nausea, somnolence, dizziness).

ropivacaine	1	3	2	May result in increased plasma levels of ropivacaine.
sevelamer	0	3	2	May result in decreased bioavailability of ciprofloxacin.
sucralfate	1	2	2	May result in decreased ciprofloxacin effectiveness.
theophylline	2	2	1	May result in elevated plasma theophylline concentrations, prolongation of theophylline elimination half-life, and theophylline toxicity (nausea, vomiting, palpitations, seizures).
tizanidine	1	1	1	May result in increased tizanidine plasma concentrations resulting in increased hypotensive and sedative effects.
warfarin	2	3	2	May result in increased risk of bleeding.
CITALOPRAM				
Anticoagulants (*abciximab, acenocoumarol, ancrod, anisindione, antithrombin III human, bivalirudin, cilostazol, clopidogrel, danaparoid, defibrotide, dermatan sulfate, dicumarol, eptifibatide, fondaparinux, lamifiban, pentosan polysulfate sodium, phenindione, phenprocoumon, sibrafiban, warfarin, xemilofiban*)	0	2	2	May result in increased risk of bleeding.

ONSET: 0 = NOT SPECIFIED, 1 = RAPID, 2 = DELAYED   SEVERITY: 1 = CONTRAINDICATED, 2 = MAJOR, 3 = MODERATE

Antiplatelet Agents (*abciximab, anagrelide, aspirin, cilostazol, clopidogrel, dipyridamole, epoprostenol, eptifibatide, iloprost, lamifiban, lexipafant, sulfinpyrazone, sulodexide, ticlopidine, tirofiban, xemilofiban*)	0	2	2	May result in increased risk of bleeding.
clorgyline	1	1	1	May result in CNS toxicity or serotonin syndrome (hypertension, hyperthermia, myoclonus, mental status changes).
clozapine	2	3	2	May result in increased risk of clozapine toxicity (sedation, seizures, hypotension).
desipramine	0	3	2	May result in possible increase in the plasma concentrations of desipramine.
dexfenfluramine	1	2	2	May result in serotonin syndrome (hypertension, hyperthermia, myoclonus, mental status changes).
fenfluramine	1	2	2	May result in serotonin syndrome (hypertension, hyperthermia, myoclonus, mental status changes).
frovatriptan	2	2	2	May result in increased risk of serotonin syndrome.
ginkgo	2	3	2	May result in increased risk of serotonin syndrome (hypertension, hyperthermia, myoclonus, mental status changes).

imipramine	1	3	2	May result in increased bioavailability and half-life of desipramine, the major metabolite of imipramine.
iproniazid	1	1	1	May result in CNS toxicity or serotonin syndrome (hypertension, hyperthermia, myoclonus, mental status changes).
irinotecan	2	3	2	May result in increased risk of myopathy or rhabdomyolysis.
isocarboxazid	1	1	1	May result in CNS toxicity or serotonin syndrome (hypertension, hyperthermia, myoclonus, mental status changes).
linezolid	1	2	2	May result in CNS toxicity or serotonin syndrome (hypertension, hyperthermia, myoclonus, mental status changes).
metoprolol	2	3	2	May result in increased metoprolol plasma concentrations and possible loss of metoprolol cardioselectivity.
moclobemide	1	1	2	May result in serotonin syndrome (hypertension, hyperthermia, myoclonus, mental status changes).
naratriptan	2	2	2	May result in increased risk of serotonin syndrome.
nialamide	1	1	1	May result in CNS toxicity or serotonin syndrome (hypertension, hyperthermia, myoclonus, mental status changes).

ONSET: 0 - NOT SPECIFIED, 1 - RAPID, 2 - DELAYED   SEVERITY: 1 - CONTRAINDICATED, 2 - MAJOR, 3 - MODERATE

NSAIDs (aceclofenac, acemetacin, alclofenac, apazone, aspirin, benoxaprofen, bromfenac, bufexamac, carprofen, celecoxib, clometacin, clonixin, dexketoprofen, diclofenac, diflunisal, dipyrone, dofetilide, droxicam, etodolac, etofenamate, felbinac, fenbufen, fenoprofen, fentiazac, floctafenine, flufenamic acid, flurbiprofen, ibuprofen, indomethacin, indoprofen, isoxicam, ketoprofen, ketorolac, lornoxicam, meclofenamate, mefanamic acid, meloxicam, nabumetone, naproxen, niflumic acid, nimesulide, oxaprozin, oxyphenbutazone, phenylbutazone, pirazolac, piroxicam, pirprofen, propyphenazon, proquazone, rofecoxib, sulindac, suprofen, tenidap, tenoxicam, tiaprofenic acid, ticrynafen, tolmetin, zomepirac)	0	3	2	May result in increased risk of bleeding.
pargyline	1	1	1	May result in CNS toxicity or serotonin syndrome (hypertension, hyperthermia, myoclonus, mental status changes).
phenelzine	1	1	1	May result in CNS toxicity or serotonin syndrome (hypertension, hyperthermia, myoclonus, mental status changes).

procarbazine	1	1	1	May result in CNS toxicity or serotonin syndrome (hypertension, hyperthermia, myoclonus, mental status changes).
rifampin	0	3	2	May result in decreased citalopram plasma concentrations with a risk of decreased citalopram efficacy.
rizatriptan	2	2	2	May result in increased risk of serotonin syndrome.
selegiline	1	1	1	May result in CNS toxicity or serotonin syndrome (hypertension, hyperthermia, myoclonus, mental status changes).
sibutramine	1	2	2	May result in increased risk of serotonin syndrome (hypertension, hyperthermia, myoclonus, mental status changes).
St. John's wort	1	2	2	May result in increased risk of serotonin syndrome (hypertension, hyperthermia, myoclonus, mental status changes).
sumatriptan	2	2	1	May result in increased risk of serotonin syndrome.
toloxatone	1	1	1	May result in CNS toxicity or serotonin syndrome (hypertension, hyperthermia, myoclonus, mental status changes).

ONSET: 0 - NOT SPECIFIED 1 - RAPID 2 - DELAYED   SEVERITY: 1 - CONTRAINDICATED 2 - MAJOR 3 - MODERATE

tranylcypromine	1	1	1	May result in CNS toxicity or serotonin syndrome (hypertension, hyperthermia, myoclonus, mental status changes).
zolmitriptan	2	2	2	May result in increased risk of serotonin syndrome.

CLARITHROMYCIN

acenocoumarol	2	3	2	May result in increased prothrombin time ratio or international normalized ratio (INR) and an increased risk of bleeding.
alfentanil	2	3	2	May result in increased plasma levels of alfentanil.
alprazolam	2	3	2	May result in increased benzodiazepine toxicity (CNS depression, ataxia, lethargy).
aprepitant	2	2	2	May result in increased plasma concentrations of aprepitant.
astemizole	2	1	2	May result in cardiotoxicity (QT prolongation, torsades de pointes, cardiac arrest).
atorvastatin	2	2	2	May result in increased atorvastatin exposure and an increased risk of myopathy or rhabdomyolysis.
bromocriptine	2	3	2	May result in increased plasma levels of bromocriptine.
carbamazepine	2	3	2	May result in increased risk of carbamazepine toxicity (ataxia, nystagmus, diplopia, headache, vomiting, apnea, seizures, coma).
cilostazol	2	3	2	May result in increased systemic exposure (AUC) of cilostazol.

Drug	Onset	Severity	Documentation	Effect
cisapride	1	1	2	May result in cardiotoxicity (QT prolongation, torsades de pointes, cardiac arrest).
colchicine	2	2	2	May result in increased plasma levels of colchicine and increased risk of toxicity.
cyclosporine	2	3	2	May result in increased risk of cyclosporine toxicity (renal dysfunction, cholestasis, paresthesias).
darunavir	0	3	1	May result in increased clarithromycin plasma concentrations.
delavirdine	2	3	2	May result in increased serum clarithromycin levels.
diazepam	2	3	2	May result in increased benzodiazepine toxicity (CNS depression, ataxia, lethargy).
digoxin	2	2	1	May result in digoxin toxicity (nausea, vomiting, arrhythmias).
disopyramide	2	2	2	May result in increased plasma levels of disopyramide; an increased risk of cardiotoxicity (QT prolongation, torsades de pointes, cardiac arrest).
efavirenz	2	3	2	May result in increased risk of rash.
ergot derivatives (*dihydroergotamine, ergoloid mesylates, ergonovine, ergotamine, methylergonovine*)	2	1	2	May result in increased risk of acute ergotism (nausea, vomiting, vasospastic ischemia).

ONSET: 0 - NOT SPECIFIED 1 - RAPID 2 - DELAYED   SEVERITY: 1 - CONTRAINDICATED 2 - MAJOR 3 - MODERATE

Drug	1	2	3	Description
estrogens (estradiol, estriol, estrone, estropipate)	0	3	2	May result in increased plasma concentrations of estrogens.
etravirine	0	2	2	May result in increased etravirine plasma concentrations; decreased clarithromycin plasma concentrations.
fentanyl	2	2	2	May result in increased or prolonged opioid effects (CNS depression, respiratory depression).
fluconazole	0	2	2	May result in increased risk of cardiotoxicity (QT prolongation, torsades de pointes, cardiac arrest).
fluoxetine	2	2	2	May result in delirium and psychosis.
gemifloxacin	0	2	2	May result in increased risk of cardiotoxicity (QT prolongation, torsades de pointes, cardiac arrest).
glipizide	1	3	2	May result in increased risk of hypoglycemia.
glyburide	1	3	1	May result in increased plasma glyburide concentrations and increased risk of hypoglycemia.
hexobarbital	2	3	2	May result in increased serum levels of hexobarbital.
indinavir	0	3	2	May result in increased clarithromycin and/or indinavir concentrations.
itraconazole	2	3	2	May result in increased itraconazole and clarithromycin concentrations.
lopinavir	2	3	2	May result in increased clarithromycin plasma concentrations and risk of side effects (diarrhea, nausea, dyspepsia).

Drug	Onset	Severity		Effect
lovastatin	2	2	2	May result in increased risk of myopathy or rhabdomyolysis.
methylprednisolone	2	3	2	May result in increased risk of steroid-induced adverse effects.
methysergide	2	1	2	May result in increased risk of acute ergotism (nausea, vomiting, vasospastic ischemia).
midazolam	2	3	2	May result in increased benzodiazepine toxicity (CNS depression, ataxia, lethargy).
nevirapine	2	3	1	May result in decreased clarithromycin concentrations.
paroxetine	2	3	2	May result in increased risk of serotonin syndrome (hypertension, hyperthermia, myoclonus, mental status changes).
phenytoin	2	3	2	May result in increased risk of phenytoin toxicity (ataxia, hyperreflexia, nystagmus, tremor).
pimozide	1	1	2	May result in increased risk of cardiotoxicity (QT prolongation, torsades de pointes, cardiac arrest).
prednisone	2	3	2	May result in increased risk of psychotic symptoms.
quinidine	1	2	1	May result in cardiotoxicity (QT prolongation, torsades de pointes, cardiac arrest).
repaglinide	0	3	2	May result in increased repaglinide exposure and plasma concentration.

ONSET: 0 = NOT SPECIFIED, 1 = RAPID, 2 = DELAYED   SEVERITY: 1 = CONTRAINDICATED, 2 = MAJOR, 3 = MODERATE

rifabutin	2	2	1	May result in subtherapeutic clarithromycin serum concentrations and increased risk of rifabutin toxicity (rash, GI disturbances, hematologic abnormalities).
rifapentine	2	3	2	May result in decreased clarithromycin effectiveness.
ritonavir	2	3	2	May result in increased clarithromycin plasma concentrations and risk of side effects (diarrhea, nausea, dyspepsia).
saquinavir	2	3	2	May result in increased saquinavir serum concentrations.
simvastatin	2	2	2	May result in increased risk of myopathy or rhabdomyolysis.
tacrolimus	2	3	2	May result in increased tacrolimus concentration and increased risk of tacrolimus toxicity (nephrotoxicity, hyperglycemia, hyperkalemia).
terfenadine	1	1	2	May result in cardiotoxicity (QT prolongation, torsades de pointes, cardiac arrest).
tipranavir	2	3	1	May result in increased exposure to both tipranavir and clarithromycin with increased risk of side effects.
tolterodine	1	3	2	May result in enhanced tolterodine bioavailability in individuals with deficient cytochrome P450 2D6 activity.
triazolam	2	3	2	May result in increased benzodiazepine toxicity (CNS depression, ataxia, lethargy).

verapamil	2	3	2	May result in increased verapamil plasma concentrations and an increased risk of hypotension and/or bradycardia.
warfarin	2	3	2	May result in increased risk of bleeding.
CLINDAMYCIN				
atracurium	1	3	2	May result in enhanced and prolonged neuromuscular blockade.
cyclosporine	2	3	2	May result in decreased cyclosporine bioavailability.
metocurine	1	3	2	May result in enhanced and prolonged neuromuscular blockade.
tubocurarine	1	3	2	May result in enhanced and prolonged neuromuscular blockade.
CLONAZEPAM				
amiodarone	2	3	2	May result in clonazepam toxicity (confusion, slurred speech, enuresis).
Barbiturates (*amobarbital, aprobarbital, butabarbital, butalbital, mephobarbital, methohexital, pentobarbital, phenobarbital, primidone, secobarbital, thiopental*)	0	2	2	May result in additive respiratory depression.

ONSET: 0 = NOT SPECIFIED 1 = RAPID 2 = DELAYED   SEVERITY: 1 = CONTRAINDICATED 2 = MAJOR 3 = MODERATE

carbamazepine	2	3	2	May result in reduced plasma levels of clonazepam.
desipramine	2	3	2	May result in decreased desipramine effectiveness.
ginkgo	2	3	2	May result in decreased anticonvulsant effectiveness.
nevirapine	0	3	2	May result in decreased plasma concentrations of clonazepam.
Opioid Analgesics (*alfentanil, anileridine, codeine, fentanyl, hydrocodone, hydromorphone, levorphanol, meperidine, morphine, morphine sulfate liposome, oxycodone, oxymorphone, propoxyphene, remifentanil, sufentanil*)	0	2	2	May result in additive respiratory depression.
ritonavir	2	3	2	May result in increased clonazepam serum concentrations and potential toxicity (excessive sedation, confusion).
St. John's wort	2	3	2	May result in reduced BZD effectiveness.
theophylline	1	3	2	May result in decreased BZD effectiveness.
CLONIDINE				
amitriptyline	2	2	2	May result in decreased antihypertensive effectiveness.
amoxapine	2	2	2	May result in decreased antihypertensive effectiveness.
atenolol	2	2	2	May result in exaggerated clonidine withdrawal response (acute hypertension).

celiprolol	2	2	2	May result in exaggerated clonidine withdrawal response (acute hypertension).
clomipramine	2	2	2	May result in decreased antihypertensive effectiveness.
cyclosporine	2	3	2	May result in increased risk of cyclosporine toxicity (renal dysfunction, cholestasis, paresthesias).
desipramine	2	2	2	May result in decreased antihypertensive effectiveness.
dothiepin	2	2	2	May result in decreased antihypertensive effectiveness.
doxepin	2	2	2	May result in decreased antihypertensive effectiveness.
fluphenazine	2	3	2	May result in increased risk of dementia.
imipramine	2	2	2	May result in decreased antihypertensive effectiveness.
labetalol	2	2	2	May result in exaggerated clonidine withdrawal response (acute hypertension).
lofepramine	2	2	2	May result in decreased antihypertensive effectiveness.
mepivacaine	1	3	2	May result in prolongation of sensory and motor block.
metoprolol	2	2	2	May result in exaggerated clonidine withdrawal response (acute hypertension).
mirtazapine	2	2	2	May result in hypertension, decreased antihypertensive effectiveness.
nadolol	2	2	2	May result in exaggerated clonidine withdrawal response (acute hypertension).

ONSET: 0 - NOT SPECIFIED, 1 - RAPID, 2 - DELAYED SEVERITY: 1 - CONTRAINDICATED, 2 - MAJOR, 3 - MODERATE

naloxone	1	3	2	May result in hypertension.
nortriptyline	2	2	2	May result in decreased antihypertensive effectiveness.
propranolol	2	2	2	May result in exaggerated clonidine withdrawal response (acute hypertension).
timolol	2	2	2	May result in exaggerated clonidine withdrawal response (acute hypertension).
trimipramine	2	2	2	May result in decreased antihypertensive effectiveness.
yohimbine	1	3	2	May result in reduced clonidine effectiveness.
CLOPIDOGREL				
amiodarone	0	3	2	May result in ineffective inhibition of platelet aggregation.
desvenlafaxine	0	2	2	May result in increased risk of bleeding.
NSAIDs (aceclofenac, acemetacin, alclofenac, apazone, benoxaprofen, bromfenac, bufexamac, carprofen, celecoxib, clometacin, clonixin, dexketoprofen, diclofenac, diflunisal, dipyrone, dofetilide, droxicam, etodolac, etofenamate, felbinac, fenbufen, fenoprofen, fentiazac, floctafenine, flufenamic acid, flurbiprofen, ibuprofen, indomethacin, indoprofen, isoxicam, ketoprofen, ketorolac, lornoxicam,	2	3	2	May result in increased risk of bleeding.

meclofenamate, mefanamic acid, meloxicam, nabumetone, naproxen, niflumic acid, nimesulide, oxaprozin, oxyphenbutazone, phenylbutazone, pirazolac, piroxicam, pirprofen, propyphenazon, proquazone, rofecoxib, sulindac, suprofen, tenidap, tenoxicam, tiaprofenic acid, ticrynafen, tolmetin, zomepirac)				
phenytoin	2	3	2	May result in increased risk of phenytoin toxicity (ataxia, hyperreflexia, nystagmus, tremor).
SSRIs (citalopram, clovoxamin, femoxetine, flexinoxan, fluoxetine, fluvoxamine, nefazodone, paroxetine, sertraline, venlafaxine, zimeldine)	0	2	2	May result in increased risk of bleeding.
venlafaxine	0	3	2	May result in increased risk of bleeding.
vitamin A	2	3	2	May result in increased risk of bleeding.
warfarin	0	2	2	May result in increased risk of bleeding.
CLOTRIMAZOLE				
Ergot Derivatives (dihydroergotamine, ergoloid mesylates, ergonovine, ergotamine, methylergonovine)	1	1	2	May result in increased risk of ergotism (nausea, vomiting, vasospastic ischemia).

ONSET: 0 - NOT SPECIFIED 1 - RAPID 2 - DELAYED   SEVERITY: 1 - CONTRAINDICATED 2 - MAJOR 3 - MODERATE

fentanyl	2	3	2	May result in increased or prolonged opioid effects (CNS depression, respiratory depression).
tacrolimus	2	3	1	May result in increased tacrolimus concentration.
trimetrexate	2	3	2	May result in increased trimetrexate toxicity (bone marrow suppression, renal & hepatic dysfunction, and gastrointestinal ulceration).
CODEINE				
Barbiturates (*amobarbital, aprobarbital, butabarbital, butalbital, mephobarbital, methohexital, pentobarbital, phenobarbital, primidone, secobarbital, thiopental*)	0	2	2	May result in additive respiratory depression.
BZDs (*adinazolam, alprazolam, bromazepam, brotizolam, chlordiazepoxide, clobazam, clonazepam, clorazepate, diazepam, estazolam, flunitrazepam, flurazepam, halazepam, ketazolam, lorazepam, lormetazepam, lormetazepam, medazepam, midazolam, nitrazepam, nordazepam, oxazepam, prazepam, temazepam, triazolam*)	0	2	2	May result in additive respiratory depression.
ethanol	1	3	2	May result in increased sedation.

	Onset	Severity	Documentation	
Muscle Relaxants, Centrally Acting (*carisoprodol, chlorzoxazone, dantrolene, mephenesin, meprobamate, metaxalone, methocarbamol*)	0	2	2	May result in additive respiratory depression.
naltrexone	1	1	2	May result in precipitation of opioid withdrawal symptoms; decreased opioid effectiveness.
Opioid Agonists/Antagonists (*buprenorphine, butorphanol, dezocine, nalbuphine, pentazocine*)	2	2	2	May result in precipitation of withdrawal symptoms (abdominal cramps, nausea, vomiting, lacrimation, rhinorrhea, anxiety, restlessness, elevation of temperature or piloerection).
COLCHICINE				
clarithromycin	2	2	2	May result in increased plasma levels of colchicine and increased risk of toxicity.
cyclosporine	2	2	2	May result in increased risk of cyclosporine toxicity (renal dysfunction, cholestasis, paresthesias); gastrointestinal dysfunction, hepatonephropathy, and neuromyopathy.
erythromycin	2	2	2	May result in increased plasma levels of colchicine and increased risk of toxicity.
fluvastatin	2	3	2	May result in increased risk of myopathy or rhabdomyolysis.

ONSET: 0 = NOT SPECIFIED 1 = RAPID 2 = DELAYED   SEVERITY: 1 = CONTRAINDICATED 2 = MAJOR 3 = MODERATE

gemfibrozil	2	2	2	May result in increased risk of myopathy or rhabdomyolysis.
grapefruit juice	2	2	2	May result in increased colchicine concentrations and increased risk for colchicine toxicity.
interferon alfa-2a	2	2	2	May result in decreased interferon alfa-2a effectiveness.
lovastatin	2	2	2	May result in increased risk of myopathy or rhabdomyolysis.
pravastatin	2	2	2	May result in increased risk of myopathy or rhabdomyolysis.
CONJUGATED ESTROGENS				
clarithromycin	0	3	2	May result in increased plasma concentrations of estrogens.
ginseng	2	3	2	May result in additive estrogenic effects.
grapefruit juice	1	3	2	May result in increased plasma concentrations of estrogens.
itraconazole	0	3	2	May result in increased plasma concentrations of estrogens.
ketoconazole	0	3	2	May result in increased plasma concentrations of estrogens.
levothyroxine	2	3	2	May result in decreased serum-free thyroxine concentration.
licorice	2	3	2	May result in increased risk of fluid retention and elevated blood pressure.
St. John's wort	0	3	2	May result in decreased plasma concentrations of estrogens and in estrogen effectiveness.

tipranavir	0	3	1	May result in decreased estrogen concentration and increased risk of developing a non-serious rash.
CYCLOBENZAPRINE				
duloxetine	0	2	2	May result in increased risk of serotonin syndrome.
fluoxetine	2	3	2	May result in increased risk of QT prolongation.
TCA measurement	1	3	1	May result in false positive TCA assay results due to structural similarity of cyclobenzaprine to the TCA class.
DESOGESTREL				
alprazolam	2	3	2	May result in increased risk of alprazolam toxicity (CNS depression, hypotension).
amprenavir	2	3	2	May result in decreased serum concentrations of amprenavir; loss of contraceptive efficacy.
bexarotene	2	3	2	May result in decreased contraceptive effectiveness.
bosentan	2	3	2	May result in decreased contraceptive effectiveness.
fosamprenavir	2	2	1	May result in decreased serum concentrations of amprenavir, altered hormonal levels, and an increased risk of hepatotoxicity.
griseofulvin	2	3	1	May result in decreased contraceptive effectiveness.
lamotrigine	2	3	2	May result in altered (increased or decreased) plasma lamotrigine concentrations.

ONSET: 0 – NOT SPECIFIED, 1 – RAPID, 2 – DELAYED   SEVERITY: CONTRAINDICATED, 2 – MAJOR, 3 – MODERATE

licorice	2	3	2	May result in increased risk of fluid retention and elevated blood pressure.
modafinil	2	3	2	May result in decreased contraceptive bioavailability and reduced contraceptive effectiveness.
prednisolone	2	3	1	May result in increased risk of corticosteroid side effects (neuropsychiatric reactions, fluid and electrolyte disturbances, hypertension, hyperglycemia).
rosuvastatin	0	3	2	May result in increased exposure to ethinyl estradiol and norgestrel.
St. John's wort	2	3	1	May result in decrease in plasma concentrations of estrogens and in contraceptive effectiveness.
topiramate	2	3	2	May result in reduced contraceptive efficacy.
DIAZEPAM				
amitriptyline	1	3	2	May result in psychomotor deficits (decreased reaction time, decreased vigilance).
amprenavir	2	3	2	May result in increased risk of diazepam toxicity (excessive sedation, confusion).
Barbiturates (*amobarbital, aprobarbital, butabarbital, butalbital, mephobarbital, methohexital, pentobarbital, phenobarbital, primidone, secobarbital, thiopental*)	0	2	2	May result in additive respiratory depression.

buprenorphine	1	2	2	May result in respiratory and cardiovascular collapse.
clarithromycin	2	3	2	May result in increased BZD toxicity (CNS depression, ataxia, lethargy).
dalfopristin	2	3	2	May result in increased risk of diazepam toxicity (excessive sedation, confusion).
disulfiram	2	3	2	May result in increased risk of CNS depression.
erythromycin	2	3	2	May result in increased BZD toxicity (CNS depression, ataxia, lethargy).
fluvoxamine	2	3	2	May result in diazepam and N-desmethyldiazepam accumulation.
fosamprenavir	2	3	2	May result in increased risk of diazepam toxicity (excessive sedation, confusion, respiratory depression).
ginkgo	2	3	2	May result in decreased anticonvulsant effectiveness.
grapefruit juice	1	3	2	May result in increased plasma concentrations of diazepam.
isoniazid	2	3	2	May result in increased risk of BZD toxicity (sedation, respiratory depression).
mirtazapine	2	3	2	May result in impairment of motor skills.

ONSET: 0 - NOT SPECIFIED, 1 - RAPID, 2 - DELAYED   SEVERITY: 1 - CONTRAINDICATED, 2 - MAJOR, 3 - MODERATE

Opioid Analgesics (*alfentanil, anileridine, codeine, fentanyl, hydrocodone, hydromorphone, levorphanol, meperidine, morphine, morphine sulfate liposome, oxycodone, oxymorphone, propoxyphene, remifentanil, sufentanil*)	0	2	2	May result in additive respiratory depression.
phenytoin	2	3	2	May result in alterations in serum phenytoin concentrations.
quinupristin	2	3	2	May result in increased risk of diazepam toxicity (excessive sedation, confusion).
rifapentine	2	3	2	May result in reduced diazepam plasma concentrations and effectiveness.
roxithromycin	2	3	2	May result in increased BZD toxicity (CNS depression, ataxia, lethargy).
St. John's wort	2	3	2	May result in reduced BZD effectiveness.
theophylline	1	3	2	May result in decreased BZD effectiveness.
troleandomycin	2	3	2	May result in increased BZD toxicity (CNS depression, ataxia, lethargy).

DICLOFENAC

ACE Inhibitors (*alacepril, benazepril, captopril, cilazapril, delapril, enalapril maleate, enalaprilat, fosinopril, imidapril, lisinopril, moexipril, pentopril,*	2	3	2	May result in decreased antihypertensive and natriuretic effects.

perindopril, quinapril, ramipril, spirapril, temocapril, trandolapril, zofenopril)				
cholestyramine	1	3	2	May result in decreased diclofenac bioavailability.
clopidogrel	2	3	2	May result in increased risk of bleeding.
colestipol	1	3	2	May result in decreased diclofenac bioavailability.
cyclosporine	2	3	2	May result in increased risk of cyclosporine toxicity (renal dysfunction, cholestasis, paresthesias).
danaparoid	1	2	2	May result in increased risk of bleeding and an increased risk of hematoma when neuraxial anesthesia is employed.
desvenlafaxine	0	2	2	May result in increased risk of bleeding.
ginkgo	2	2	2	May result in increased risk of bleeding.
lithium	2	3	2	May result in lithium toxicity (weakness, tremor, excessive thirst, confusion).
LMWHs (*ardeparin, certoparin, dalteparin, enoxaparin, nadroparin, parnaparin, reviparin, tinzaparin*)	1	2	2	May result in increased risk of bleeding.
Loop Diuretics (*azosemide, bumetanide, ethacrynic acid, furosemide, piretanide, torsemide*)	2	3	2	May result in decreased diuretic and antihypertensive efficacy.

ONSET: 0 = NOT SPECIFIED 1 = RAPID 2 = DELAYED   SEVERITY: 1 = CONTRAINDICATED 2 = MAJOR 3 = MODERATE

methotrexate	2	2	2	May result in methotrexate toxicity (leukopenia, thrombocytopenia, anemia, nephrotoxicity, mucosal ulcerations).
Potassium-Sparing Diuretics (*amiloride, canrenoate, eplerenone, spironolactone, triamterene, torsemide*)	2	3	2	May result in reduced diuretic effectiveness, hyperkalemia, or possible nephrotoxicity.
SSRIs (*citalopram, clovoxamine, femoxetine, fleinoxan, fluoxetine, nefazodone, paroxetine, sertraline, venlafaxine, zimeldine*)	0	3	2	May result in increased risk of bleeding.
Sulfonylureas (*acetohexamide, chlorpropamide, gliclazide, glimepride, glipizide, gliquidone, glyburide, tolazamide, tolbutamide*)	2	3	2	May result in increased risk of hypoglycemia.
tacrolimus	2	2	2	May result in acute renal failure.
Thiazide Diuretics (*bemetizide, bendroflumethiazide, benzthiazide, buthiazide, chlorthiazide, chlorthalidone, clopamide, cyclopenthiazide, cyclothiazide, HCTZ, hydroflumethiazide, indapamide, methyclothiazide, metolazone, polythiazide, quinethazone, trichlormethiazide, xipamide*)	2	3	2	May result in decreased diuretic and antihypertensive efficacy.

venlafaxine	0	3	2	May result in increased risk of bleeding.

DICYCLOMINE

betel nut	2	3	2	May result in reduced anticholinergic effect of dicyclomine.

DIGOXIN

acarbose	2	3	2	May result in decreased digoxin efficacy.
alprazolam	2	2	2	May result in digoxin toxicity (nausea, vomiting, arrhythmias).
aminosalicylic acid	1	3	2	May result in reduced digoxin serum concentrations.
amiodarone	2	2	1	May result in digoxin toxicity (nausea, vomiting, cardiac arrhythmias).
Antacids (*aluminum carbonate, basic, aluminum hydroxide, aluminum phosphate, dihydroxyaluminum aminoacetate, dihydroxyaluminum sodium carbonate, fludrocortisone, fluocortolone, hydrocortisone, magaldrate, magnesium carbonate, magnesium hydroxide, magnesium oxide, magnesium trisilicate*)	1	3	2	May result in decreased digoxin levels.
arbutamine	1	3	2	May result in unreliable arbutamine test results.
atorvastatin	2	3	2	May result in increased plasma concentrations of digoxin.

ONSET: 0 - NOT SPECIFIED 1 - RAPID 2 - DELAYED   SEVERITY: 1 - CONTRAINDICATED 2 - MAJOR 3 - MODERATE

azithromycin	2	3	2	May result in digoxin toxicity (vomiting, cardiac arrhythmias).
azosemide	2	3	2	May result in digoxin toxicity (nausea, vomiting, cardiac arrhythmias).
β-Blockers (acebutolol, alprenolol, atenolol, betaxolol, bevantolol, bisoprolol, bucindolol, carteolol, carvedilol, celiprolol, dilevalol, esmolol, labetalol, levobunolol, mepindolol, metipranolol, metoprolol, nadolol, nebivolol, oxprenolol, penbutolol, pindolol, propranolol, sotalol, talinolol, tertatolol, timolol)	2	3	2	May result in AV block and possible digoxin toxicity.
bepridil	2	3	2	May result in digoxin toxicity (nausea, vomiting, arrhythmias).
buthiazide	2	2	1	May result in digitalis toxicity (nausea, vomiting, arrhythmias).
calcium	1	2	2	May result in serious risk of arrhythmia and cardiovascular collapse.
canrenoate	1	3	2	May result in increased cardiac contractility.
cascara sagrada	2	3	2	May result in hypokalemia secondary to cascara sagrada bark intake, which may increase the risk of digoxin toxicity.
cholestyramine	1	3	2	May result in decreased digoxin levels.
clarithromycin	2	2	1	May result in digoxin toxicity (nausea, vomiting, arrhythmias).

colestipol	1	3	2	May result in decreased digoxin effectiveness.
conivaptan	0	2	2	May result in increased digoxin plasma concentrations and increased risk of digoxin toxicity (nausea, vomiting, arrhythmias).
cyclosporine	2	3	2	May result in digoxin toxicity (nausea, vomiting, cardiac arrhythmias).
diltiazem	2	3	2	May result in increased serum digoxin concentrations and toxicity (nausea, vomiting, arrhythmias).
disopyramide	2	3	2	May result in digoxin toxicity (nausea, vomiting, cardiac arrhythmias).
erythromycin	2	2	2	May result in increased digoxin levels and digoxin toxicity (nausea, vomiting, arrhythmias).
flecainide	2	3	2	May result in digoxin toxicity (nausea, vomiting, cardiac arrhythmias).
fluoxetine	2	3	2	May result in increased risk of digoxin toxicity (nausea, vomiting, arrhythmias).
food	1	3	2	May result in decreased peak digoxin concentrations.
furosemide	2	3	2	May result in digoxin toxicity (nausea, vomiting, cardiac arrhythmias).
gatifloxacin	2	3	2	May result in increased risk of digoxin toxicity (nausea, vomiting, arrhythmias).

ONSET: 0 - NOT SPECIFIED, 1 - RAPID, 2 - DELAYED   SEVERITY: 1 - CONTRAINDICATED, 2 - MAJOR, 3 - MODERATE

hydroxychloroquine	2	3	2	May result in increased serum digoxin concentrations.
indecainide	2	3	2	May result in digoxin toxicity (nausea, vomiting, arrhythmias).
indomethacin	2	2	2	May result in increased risk of digoxin toxicity (nausea, vomiting, cardiac arrhythmias).
itraconazole	2	2	2	May result in increased risk of digoxin toxicity (nausea, vomiting, arrhythmias).
kyushin	1	2	2	May result in increased risk of digoxin toxicity.
lenalidomide	0	3	2	May result in increased digoxin plasma concentrations.
lornoxicam	2	3	2	May result in digoxin toxicity (nausea, vomiting, arrhythmias).
metoclopramide	2	3	2	May result in decreased digoxin levels.
mibefradil	2	3	2	May result in increased risk of digoxin toxicity (nausea, vomiting, arrhythmias).
nefazodone	2	3	2	May result in increased digoxin serum concentrations and possibly increase the risk of digoxin toxicity (nausea, vomiting, cardiac arrhythmias).
neomycin	2	3	2	May result in decreased digoxin levels.
nilvadipine	2	3	2	May result in increased serum digoxin concentrations and toxicity (nausea, vomiting, arrhythmias).
nisoldipine	2	3	2	May result in digoxin toxicity (nausea, vomiting, arrhythmias).
nitrendipine	2	3	2	May result in increased serum digoxin concentrations and toxicity (nausea, vomiting, arrhythmias).

	Onset	Severity		
omeprazole	1	3	2	May result in increased risk of digoxin toxicity (nausea, vomiting, arrhythmias).
pancuronium	1	3	1	May result in increased risk of cardiac arrhythmias.
paromomycin	1	3	2	May result in reduced digoxin serum concentrations and efficacy.
piretanide	2	3	2	May result in digoxin toxicity (nausea, vomiting, cardiac arrhythmias).
propafenone	2	2	2	May result in digoxin toxicity (nausea, vomiting, cardiac arrhythmias).
propantheline	1	2	2	May result in increased serum digoxin levels.
quinidine	2	2	1	May result in digoxin toxicity (nausea, vomiting, cardiac arrhythmias).
quinine	2	2	2	May result in digoxin toxicity (nausea, vomiting, cardiac arrhythmias).
rabeprazole	2	3	2	May result in increased risk of digoxin toxicity (nausea, vomiting, arrhythmias).
ranolazine	0	3	2	May result in increased digoxin steady-state plasma concentrations.
rifampin	2	3	1	May result in decreased digoxin levels.
rifapentine	2	3	2	May result in decreased cardiac glycoside effectiveness.

ONSET: 0 – NOT SPECIFIED 1 – RAPID 2 – DELAYED   SEVERITY: 1 – CONTRAINDICATED 2 – MAJOR 3 – MODERATE

ritonavir	2	2	2	May result in increased digoxin plasma concentrations and increased risk of digoxin toxicity (nausea, vomiting, arrhythmias).
roxithromycin	2	3	2	May result in possible digoxin toxicity (nausea, vomiting, arrhythmias).
simvastatin	2	3	2	May result in increased risk of digoxin toxicity (nausea, vomiting, arrhythmias).
spironolactone	2	2	2	May result in digoxin toxicity (nausea, vomiting, cardiac arrhythmias).
St. John's wort	2	2	2	May result in reduced digoxin efficacy.
sucralfate	2	3	2	May result in decreased digoxin effectiveness.
sulfasalazine	1	3	2	May result in decreased digoxin levels.
telithromycin	2	3	2	May result in increased digoxin plasma levels.
telmisartan	2	3	2	May result in increased risk of digoxin toxicity (nausea, vomiting, arrhythmias).
tetracycline	2	2	2	May result in increased digoxin levels and digoxin toxicity (nausea, vomiting, cardiac arrhythmias).
Thiazide Diuretics (bemetizide, bendroflumethiazide, benzthiazide, buthiazide, chlorthiazide, chlorthalidone, clopamide, cyclopenthiazide, cyclothiazide, HCTZ, hydroflumethiazide,	2	2	1	May result in digitalis toxicity (nausea, vomiting, arrhythmias).

indapamide, methyclothiazide, metolazone, polythiazide, quinethazone, trichlormethiazide, xipamide)				
torsemide	2	3	2	May result in digoxin toxicity (nausea, vomiting, cardiac arrhythmias).
tramadol	2	3	2	May result in increased risk of digoxin toxicity (nausea, vomiting, cardiac arrhythmias).
trazodone	2	3	2	May result in increased digoxin serum concentrations and an increased risk of digoxin toxicity (nausea, vomiting, arrhythmias).
trimethoprim	2	3	2	May result in increased risk of digoxin toxicity.
valspodar	1	3	2	May result in increased risk of digoxin toxicity (nausea, vomiting, arrhythmias).
verapamil	2	2	1	May result in increased serum digoxin concentrations and toxicity (nausea, vomiting, arrhythmias).
DILTIAZEM				
alfentanil	1	3	1	May result in prolonged alfentanil efficacy.
alfuzosin	0	3	2	May result in increased alfuzosin exposure.
amiodarone	1	2	2	May result in bradycardia, atrioventricular block and/or sinus arrest.
aprepitant	2	2	2	May result in increased plasma concentrations of aprepitant.

ONSET: 0 - NOT SPECIFIED, 1 - RAPID, 2 - DELAYED   SEVERITY: 1 - CONTRAINDICATED, 2 - MAJOR, 3 - MODERATE,

aspirin	2	3	2	May result in prolongation of bleeding time.
atazanavir	0	2	1	May result in increased risk of cardiotoxicity (prolonged PR interval).
atorvastatin	2	2	2	May result in increased risk of rhabdomyolysis.
β-Blockers (acebutolol, alprenolol, atenolol, betaxolol, bevantolol, bisoprolol, bucindolol, carteolol, carvedilol, celiprolol, dilevalol, esmolol, labetalol, levobunolol, mepindolol, metipranolol, metoprolol, nadolol, nebivolol, oxprenolol, penbutolol, pindolol, propranolol, sotalol, talinolol, tertatolol, timolol)	1	3	2	May result in increased risk of hypotension, bradycardia, AV conduction disturbances.
buspirone	1	3	2	May result in increased risk of enhanced buspirone effects.
carbamazepine	2	3	2	May result in carbamazepine toxicity (ataxia, nystagmus, diplopia, headache, vomiting, apnea, seizures, coma).
celecoxib	2	3	2	May result in loss of blood pressure control.
cilostazol	2	3	2	May result in increased risk of cilostazol adverse effects (headache, diarrhea, abnormal stools).
cimetidine	1	3	2	May result in increased diltiazem concentrations and possible cardiovascular toxicity.

cisapride	2	1	2	May result in increased risk of cardiotoxicity (QT prolongation, torsades de pointes, cardiac arrest).
colestipol	1	3	2	May result in decreased diltiazem bioavailability.
cyclosporine	2	3	2	May result in increased risk of cyclosporine toxicity (renal dysfunction, cholestasis, paresthesias).
dalfopristin	2	3	2	May result in increased risk of diltiazem toxicity (dizziness, headache, flushing, peripheral edema).
digitoxin	2	3	2	May result in increased serum digitoxin concentrations or toxicity (nausea, vomiting, cardiac arrhythmias).
digoxin	2	3	2	May result in increased serum digoxin concentrations and toxicity (nausea, vomiting, arrhythmias).
dutasteride	0	3	2	May result in increased dutasteride plasma concentrations.
efavirenz	0	3	1	May result in significantly decreased exposures and plasma concentrations of diltiazem and its metabolites.
enflurane	1	3	2	May result in cardiac toxicity (bradycardia, asystole).
erythromycin	0	2	2	May result in increased risk of cardiotoxicity (QT prolongation, torsades de pointes, cardiac arrest).
fentanyl	1	2	2	May result in severe hypotension.
food	1	3	2	May result in increased plasma concentrations.

ONSET: 0 – NOT SPECIFIED 1 – RAPID 2 – DELAYED   SEVERITY: 1 – CONTRAINDICATED 2 – MAJOR 3 – MODERATE

fosphenytoin	2	3	2	May result in increased risk of phenytoin toxicity (ataxia, hyperreflexia, nystagmus, tremor).
guggul	1	3	2	May result in reduced diltiazem effectiveness.
indinavir	0	3	2	May result in increased plasma concentrations of CCB.
lithium	2	3	2	May result in neurotoxicity, psychosis.
lovastatin	1	3	2	May result in increased plasma concentrations of lovastatin and increased risk of myopathy or rhabdomyolysis.
methylprednisolone	1	3	2	May result in increased methylprednisolone plasma concentrations and enhanced adrenal-suppressant effects.
midazolam	1	3	2	May result in increased/prolonged sedation.
moricizine	2	3	2	May result in increased moricizine concentrations and decreased diltiazem concentrations.
nevirapine	0	3	2	May result in decreased plasma concentrations of diltiazem.
nifedipine	1	3	2	May result in nifedipine toxicity (headache, peripheral edema, hypotension, tachycardia).
phenytoin	2	3	2	May result in increased risk of phenytoin toxicity (ataxia, hyperreflexia, nystagmus, tremor).
quinupristin	2	3	2	May result in increased risk of diltiazem toxicity (dizziness, headache, flushing, peripheral edema).

ranolazine	0	1	2	May result in increased ranolazine steady-state plasma concentrations and an increased risk of cardiotoxicity (QT prolongation, torsades de pointes, cardiac arrest).
rifampin	2	3	2	May result in decreased diltiazem effectiveness.
rifapentine	2	3	2	May result in decreased CCB effectiveness.
ritonavir	2	3	2	May result in increased diltiazem serum concentrations and potential toxicity (dizziness, headache, flushing, peripheral edema, hypotension, cardiac arrhythmias).
saquinavir	1	3	2	May result in increased risk of diltiazem toxicity (dizziness, headache, flushing, peripheral edema, hypotension, cardiac arrhythmias).
simvastatin	1	3	1	May result in increased serum concentration of simvastatin.
sirolimus	2	3	2	May result in increased risk of sirolimus toxicity (anemia, leukopenia, thrombocytopenia, hypokalemia, diarrhea).
St. John's wort	2	3	2	May result in reduced bioavailability of CCB.
tacrolimus	2	3	2	May result in increased tacrolimus concentration.
triazolam	1	3	2	May result in increased serum triazolam levels and increased intensity of sedation.
voriconazole	0	3	2	May result in increased plasma concentrations of CCB.

ONSET: 0 - NOT SPECIFIED 1 - RAPID 2 - DELAYED   SEVERITY: 1 - CONTRAINDICATED 2 - MAJOR 3 - MODERATE

DOXAZOSIN

β-Blockers (acebutolol, alprenolol, atenolol, betaxolol, bevantolol, bisoprolol, bucindolol, carteolol, carvedilol, celiprolol, dilevalol, esmolol, labetalol, levobunolol, mepindolol, metipranolol, metoprolol, nadolol, nebivolol, oxprenolol, penbutolol, pindolol, propranolol, sotalol, talinolol, tertatolol, timolol)	1	3	2	May result in exaggerated hypotensive response to the first dose of the α-blocker.
nifedipine	2	3	2	May result in increased plasma concentration of nifedipine which may result in increased risk of hypotension.
sildenafil	1	3	2	May result in potentiation of hypotensive effects.
tadalafil	1	2	2	May result in potentiation of hypotensive effects.
vardenafil	1	2	1	May result in potentiation of hypotensive effects.

DOXYCYCLINE

Aluminum, Calcium, or Magnesium Containing Products (aluminum carbonate, basic, aluminum hydroxide, aluminum phosphate, calcium, dihydroxyaluminum aminoacetate, dihydroxyaluminum sodium carbonate, magaldrate, magnesium carbonate,	1	3	2	May result in decreased effectiveness of tetracyclines.

Drug	Onset	Severity		Description
magnesium hydroxide, magnesium oxide, magnesium trisilicate)				
bismuth subsalicylate	2	3	2	May result in decreased doxycycline effectiveness.
Contraceptives, Combination (*ethinyl estradiol, mestranol, norelgestromin, norethindrone, norgestrel*)	2	3	2	May result in decreased contraceptive effectiveness.
fosphenytoin	2	3	2	May result in decreased doxycycline effectiveness.
iron	2	3	2	May result in decreased tetracycline and iron effectiveness.
isotretinoin	2	2	2	May result in pseudotumor cerebri (benign intracranial hypertension).
methotrexate	1	2	2	May result in increased risk of methotrexate toxicity (leukopenia, thrombocytopenia, anemia, nephrotoxicity, mucosal ulcerations.
Penicillins (*penicillin g, penicillin g procaine, penicillin v*)	2	3	2	May result in decreased antibacterial effectiveness.
rifampin	2	3	2	May result in reduced doxycycline serum concentrations and potential loss of doxycycline efficacy.
rifapentine	2	3	2	May result in decreased doxycycline effectiveness.
DROSPIRENONE				
alprazolam	2	2	2	May result in increased risk of alprazolam toxicity (CNS depression, hypotension).

ONSET: 0 - NOT SPECIFIED, 1 - RAPID, 2 - DELAYED   SEVERITY: 1 - CONTRAINDICATED, 2 - MAJOR, 3 - MODERATE

amprenavir	2	3	2	May result in decreased serum concentrations of amprenavir; loss of contraceptive efficacy.
bexarotene	2	3	2	May result in decreased contraceptive effectiveness.
bosentan	2	3	2	May result in decreased contraceptive effectiveness.
fosamprenavir	2	2	1	May result in decreased serum concentrations of amprenavir, altered hormonal levels, and an increased risk of hepatotoxicity.
lamotrigine	2	3	2	May result in altered (increased or decreased) plasma lamotrigine concentrations.
prednisolone	2	3	1	May result in increased risk of corticosteroid side effects (neuropsychiatric reactions, fluid and electrolyte disturbances, hypertension, hyperglycemia).
DULOXETINE				
Antiarrhythmic Agents, Class IC (*cifenline, encainide, flecainide, indecainide, lorcainide, propafenone, recainam*)	0	2	2	May result in increased class IC antiarrhythmic serum concentrations and increased risk of cardiotoxicity (QT prolongation, torsades de pointes, cardiac arrest).
Anticoagulants (*abciximab, acenocoumarol, ancrod, anisindione, antithrombin III human, bivalirudin, cilostazol, clopidogrel, danaparoid, defibrotide, dermatan sulfate, dicumarol, eptifibatide, fondaparinux,*	0	2	2	May result in increased risk of bleeding.

lamifiban, pentosan polysulfate sodium, phenindione, phenprocoumon, sibrafiban, warfarin, xemilofiban)				
Antiplatelet Agents (abciximab, anagrelide, aspirin, cilostazol, clopidogrel, dipyridamole, epoprostenol, eptifibatide, iloprost, lamifiban, lexipafant, sulfinpyrazone, sulodexide, ticlopidine, tirofiban, xemilofiban)	0	2	2	May result in increased risk of bleeding.
enoxacin	0	3	2	May result in increased duloxetine bioavailability and risk of adverse effects.
fluoxetine	0	3	2	May result in increased duloxetine and fluoxetine serum concentrations and risk of adverse effects.
fluvoxamine	0	3	2	May result in increased duloxetine bioavailability and risk of adverse effects.
linezolid	1	2	2	May result in CNS toxicity or serotonin syndrome (hypertension, hyperthermia, myoclonus, mental status changes).
MAOIs (clorgyline, isocarboxazid, lazabemide, moclobemide, nialamide, pargyline, phenelzine, rasagline, selegiline, toloxatone, tranylcypromine)	1	1	2	May result in CNS toxicity or serotonin syndrome (hypertension, hyperthermia, myoclonus, mental status changes).

ONSET: 0 = NOT SPECIFIED, 1 = RAPID, 2 = DELAYED   SEVERITY: 1 = CONTRAINDICATED, 2 = MAJOR, 3 = MODERATE

NSAIDs (aceclofenac, acemetacin, alclofenac, apazone, aspirin, benoxaprofen, bromfenac, bufexamac, carprofen, celecoxib, clometacin, clonixin, dexketoprofen, diclofenac, diflunisal, dipyrone, dofetilide, droxicam, etodolac, etofenamate, felbinac, fenbufen, fenoprofen, fentiazac, floctafenine, flufenamic acid, flurbiprofen, ibuprofen, indomethacin, indoprofen, isoxicam, ketoprofen, ketorolac, lornoxicam, meclofenamate, mefenamic acid, meloxicam, nabumetone, naproxen, niflumic acid, nimesulide, oxaprozin, oxyphenbutazone, phenylbutazone, pirazolac, piroxicam, pirprofen, propyphenazon, proquazone, rofecoxib, sulindac, suprofen, tenidap, tenoxicam, tiaprofenic acid, ticrynafen, tolmetin, zomepirac)	0	3	2	May result in increased risk of bleeding.
paroxetine	0	3	2	May result in increased duloxetine and paroxetine serum concentrations and risk of adverse effects.
Phenothiazines (acetophenazine, chlorpromazine, dixyrazine, ethopropazine, fluphenazine,	0	3	2	May result in increased phenothiazine serum concentrations and potential toxicity (sedation, confusion, cardiac arrhythmias, orthostatic hypotension, hyperthermia,

mesoridazine, methdilazine, methotrimeprazine, metopimazine, perazine, periciazine, perphenazine, pipotiazine, prochlorperazine, promazine, promethazine, propiomazine, thiethylperazine, thiopropazate, thioproperazine, trifluoperazine, triflupromazine, trimeprazine)				extrapyramidal effects).
quinidine	0	3	2	May result in increased duloxetine serum concentrations and risk of adverse effects.
TCAs (amineptine, amitriptyline, amitriptylinoxide, amoxapine, clomipramine, desipramine, dibenzepin, dothiepin, doxepin, imipramine, lofepramine, melitracen, nortriptyline, opipramol, protriptyline, tianeptine, trimipramine)	0	3	2	May result in increased TCA serum concentrations and potential toxicity (anticholinergic effects, sedation, confusion, cardiac arrhythmias).
thioridazine	0	1	2	May result in increased thioridazine serum concentrations and risk of cardiac arrhythmia.
warfarin	2	2	2	May result in increased INR and increased risk of bleeding.
DUTASTERIDE				
cimetidine	0	3	2	May result in increase in dutasteride plasma concentrations.

ONSET: 0 = NOT SPECIFIED, 1 = RAPID, 2 = DELAYED   SEVERITY: 1 = CONTRAINDICATED, 2 = MAJOR, 3 = MODERATE

ciprofloxacin	0	3	2	May result in increase in dutasteride plasma concentrations.
diltiazem	0	3	2	May result in increase in dutasteride plasma concentrations.
ketoconazole	0	3	2	May result in increase in dutasteride plasma concentrations.
ritonavir	0	3	2	May result in increase in dutasteride plasma concentrations.
verapamil	0	3	2	May result in increase in dutasteride plasma concentrations.
ENALAPRIL				
aliskiren	0	3	2	May result in hyperkalemia.
bupivacaine	2	3	2	May result in bradycardia and hypotension with loss of consciousness.
capsaicin	1	3	2	May result in increased risk of cough.
digoxin measurement	0	3	2	May result in false decreases in serum digoxin level due to unknown mechanism.
lithium	2	3	2	May result in lithium toxicity (weakness, tremor, excessive thirst, confusion) and/or nephrotoxicity.
Loop Diuretics (azosemide, bumetanide, ethacrynic acid, furosemide, piretanide, torsemide)	1	3	2	May result in postural hypotension (first dose).
nesiritide	2	3	2	May result in increased symptomatic hypotension.
NSAIDs (aceclofenac, acemetacin, alclofenac, apazone, aspirin, benoxaprofen, bromfenac, bufexamac,	2	3	2	May result in decreased antihypertensive and natriuretic effects.

carprofen, celecoxib, clometacin, clonixin, dexketoprofen, diclofenac, diflunisal, dipyrone, dofetilide, droxicam, etodolac, etofenamate, felbinac, fenbufen, fenoprofen, fentiazac, floctafenine, flufenamic acid, flurbiprofen, ibuprofen, indomethacin, indoprofen, isoxicam, ketoprofen, ketorolac, lornoxicam, meclofenamate, mefanamic acid, meloxicam, nabumetone, naproxen, niflumic acid, nimesulide, oxaprozin, oxyphenbutazone, phenylbutazone, pirazolac, piroxicam, pirprofen, propyphenazon, proquazone, rofecoxib, sulindac, suprofen, tenidap, tenoxicam, tiaprofenic acid, ticrynafen, tolmetin, zomepirac)				
potassium	2	2	2	May result in hyperkalemia.
Potassium-Sparing Diuretics (amiloride, canrenoate, eplerenone, spironolactone, triamterene, torsemide)	2	2	2	May result in hyperkalemia.

Thiazide Diuretics (*bemetizide, bendroflumethiazide, benzthiazide, buthiazide, chlorthiazide, chlorthalidone, clopamide, cyclopenthiazide, cyclothiazide, HCTZ, hydroflumethiazide, indapamide, methyclothiazide, metolazone, polythiazide, quinethazone, trichlormethiazide, xipamide*)	1	3	2	May result in postural hypotension (first dose).

ESCITALOPRAM

Anticoagulants (*abciximab, acenocoumarol, ancrod, anisindione, antithrombin III human, bivalirudin, cilostazol, clopidogrel, danaparoid, defibrotide, dermatan sulfate, dicumarol, eptifibatide, fondaparinux, lamifiban, pentosan polysulfate sodium, phenindione, phenprocoumon, sibrafiban, warfarin, xemilofiban*)	0	2	2	May result in increased risk of bleeding.
cimetidine	2	3	2	May result in increased bioavailability of escitalopram.
desipramine	0	3	2	May result in increased bioavailability and plasma concentrations of desipramine.
eletriptan	2	2	2	May result in increased risk of serotonin syndrome.

frovatriptan	2	2	2	May result in increased risk of serotonin syndrome.
ginkgo	2	3	2	May result in increased risk of serotonin syndrome (hypertension, hyperthermia, myoclonus, mental status changes).
hydrocodone	2	3	2	May result in increased risk of serotonin syndrome (tachycardia, hyperthermia, myoclonus, mental status changes).
ketoconazole	0	3	2	May result in decreased ketoconazole bioavailability.
lamotrigine	2	3	2	May result in increased risk of myoclonus.
lithium	2	3	1	May result in possible increased lithium concentrations and/or an increased risk of SSRI-related serotonin syndrome (hypertension, hyperthermia, myoclonus, mental status changes).
metoprolol	2	3	2	May result in increased metoprolol plasma concentrations and possible loss of metoprolol cardioselectivity.
naratriptan	2	2	2	May result in increased risk of serotonin syndrome.

NSAIDs (aceclofenac, acemetacin, alclofenac, apazone, aspirin, benoxaprofen, bromfenac, bufexamac, carprofen, celecoxib, clometacin, clonixin, dexketoprofen, diclofenac, diflunisal, dipyrone, dofetilide, droxicam, etodolac, etofenamate, felbinac, fenbufen, fenoprofen, fentiazac, floctafenine, flufenamic acid, flurbiprofen, ibuprofen, indomethacin, indoprofen, isoxicam, ketoprofen, ketorolac, lornoxicam, meclofenamate, mefanamic acid, meloxicam, nabumetone, naproxen, niflumic acid, nimesulide, oxaprozin, oxyphenbutazone, phenylbutazone, pirazolac, piroxicam, pirprofen, propyphenazon, proquazone, rofecoxib, sulindac, suprofen, tenidap, tenoxicam, tiaprofenic acid, ticrynafen, tolmetin, zomepirac)	0	3	2	May result in increased risk of bleeding.
oxycodone	2	2	2	May result in increased risk of serotonin syndrome (tachycardia, hyperthermia, myoclonus, mental status changes).
rizatriptan	2	2	2	May result in increased risk of serotonin syndrome.

sibutramine	1	2	2	May result in increased risk of serotonin syndrome (hypertension, hyperthermia, myoclonus, mental status changes).
St. John's wort	1	2	2	May result in increased risk of serotonin syndrome (hypertension, hyperthermia, myoclonus, mental status changes).
sumatriptan	2	2	2	May result in increased risk of serotonin syndrome.
zolmitriptan	2	2	2	May result in increased risk of serotonin syndrome.
ESOMEPRAZOLE				
atazanavir	0	2	2	May result in decreased atazanavir plasma concentrations and risk of diminished therapeutic effect of atazanavir.
cranberry	1	3	2	May result in reduced effectiveness of proton pump inhibitors.
warfarin	2	3	2	May result in elevations in INR serum values and potentiation of anticoagulation effects.
ESTRADIOL				
clarithromycin	0	3	2	May result in increased plasma concentrations of estrogens.
ginseng	2	3	2	May result in additive estrogenic effects.
grapefruit juice	1	3	2	May result in increased plasma concentrations of estrogens.
itraconazole	0	3	2	May result in increased plasma concentrations of estrogens.

ONSET: 0 - UNSPECIFIED, 1 - RAPID, 2 - DELAYED   SEVERITY: 1 - CONTRAINDICATED, 2 - MAJOR, 3 - MODERATE

ketoconazole	0	3	2	May result in increased plasma concentrations of estrogens.
levothyroxine	2	3	2	May result in decreased serum-free thyroxine concentration.
licorice	2	3	2	May result in increased risk of fluid retention and elevated blood pressure.
St. John's wort	0	3	2	May result in decreased plasma concentrations of estrogens and in estrogen effectiveness.
tacrine	2	3	2	May result in increased risk of tacrine adverse effects.
tipranavir	0	3	1	May result in decreased estrogen concentration and increased risk of developing a non-serious rash.
ESZOPICLONE				
ethanol	1	3	2	May result in impaired psychomotor functions and risk of increased sedation.
ketoconazole	0	3	2	May result in increased plasma concentrations of eszopiclone.
ETHINYL ESTRADIOL				
alprazolam	2	3	2	May result in increased risk of alprazolam toxicity (CNS depression, hypotension).
amoxicillin	2	3	2	May result in decreased contraceptive effectiveness.
ampicillin	2	3	2	May result in decreased contraceptive effectiveness.

Drug	Onset	Severity	Documentation	Effect
amprenavir	2	3	2	May result in decreased serum concentrations of amprenavir; loss of contraceptive efficacy.
aprepitant	2	3	2	May result in reduced efficacy of combination contraceptives.
bacampicillin	2	3	2	May result in decreased contraceptive effectiveness.
betamethasone	2	3	2	May result in increased corticosteroid effects.
bexarotene	2	3	2	May result in decreased contraceptive effectiveness.
bosentan	2	3	2	May result in decreased contraceptive effectiveness.
caffeine	1	3	2	May result in enhanced CNS stimulation.
carbamazepine	2	3	2	May result in decreased plasma concentrations of estrogens and in estrogen effectiveness.
colesevelam	1	3	2	May result in decreased contraceptive effectiveness.
cyclosporine	2	3	2	May result in increased risk of cyclosporine toxicity (renal dysfunction, cholestasis, paresthesias).
doxycycline	2	3	2	May result in decreased contraceptive effectiveness.
felbamate	2	2	2	May result in decreased contraceptive effectiveness and intermenstrual bleeding.
fosamprenavir	2	2	1	May result in decreased serum concentrations of amprenavir, altered hormonal levels, and an increased risk of hepatotoxicity.

ONSET: 0 - NOT SPECIFIED 1 - RAPID 2 - DELAYED   SEVERITY: 1 - CONTRAINDICATED 2 - MAJOR 3 - MODERATE

INTERACTING DRUG	ONSET	SEVERITY	EVIDENCE	WARNING
fosaprepitant	2	3	2	May result in reduced efficacy of combination contraceptives.
fosphenytoin	2	3	2	May result in decreased contraceptive effectiveness.
ginseng	2	3	2	May result in additive estrogenic effects.
grapefruit juice	1	3	2	May result in increased plasma concentrations of estrogens.
griseofulvin	2	3	1	May result in decreased contraceptive effectiveness.
lamotrigine	2	3	2	May result in altered (increased or decreased) plasma lamotrigine concentrations.
licorice	2	3	2	May result in increased risk of fluid retention and elevated blood pressure.
minocycline	2	3	2	May result in decreased contraceptive efficacy.
modafinil	2	3	2	May result in decreased contraceptive bioavailability and reduced contraceptive effectiveness.
mycophenolate mofetil	0	3	2	May result in decreased contraceptive exposure.
mycophenolic acid	1	3	2	May result in decreased levonorgestrel exposure.
nelfinavir	2	3	2	May result in contraceptive failure.
nevirapine	2	3	2	May result in loss of contraceptive efficacy.
oxcarbazepine	2	3	2	May result in decreased contraceptive effectiveness.
oxytetracycline	2	3	2	May result in decreased contraceptive effectiveness.

phenobarbital	2	3	2	May result in decreased plasma concentrations of estrogens and in contraceptive effectiveness.
phenytoin	2	3	2	May result in decreased contraceptive effectiveness.
pioglitazone	2	3	2	May result in loss of contraceptive efficacy.
prednisolone	2	3	1	May result in increased risk of corticosteroid side effects (neuropsychiatric reactions, fluid and electrolyte disturbances, hypertension, hyperglycemia).
primidone	2	3	2	May result in decreased contraceptive effectiveness.
rifabutin	2	3	2	May result in increased risk of contraceptive failure.
rifampin	2	3	1	May result in decreased plasma concentrations of estrogens and in contraceptive effectiveness.
rifapentine	2	3	2	May result in loss of oral contraceptive efficacy.
ritonavir	2	3	2	May result in altered contraceptive effectiveness and risk of side effects.
rosuvastatin	0	3	2	May result in increased exposure to ethinyl estradiol and norgestrel.
selegiline	1	3	2	May result in increased selegiline oral bioavailability and an increased risk of selegiline adverse reactions.
St. John's wort	2	3	1	May result in decreased plasma concentrations of estrogens and in contraceptive effectiveness.

ONSET: 0 - NOT SPECIFIED 1 - RAPID 2 - DELAYED   SEVERITY: 1 - CONTRAINDICATED 2 - MAJOR 3 - MODERATE

tetracycline	2	3	2	May result in decreased contraceptive effectiveness.
tipranavir	0	3	1	May result in decreased estrogen concentration and increased risk of developing a non-serious rash.
tizanidine	1	2	2	May result in increased tizanidine plasma concentrations resulting in increased hypotensive and sedative effects.
topiramate	2	3	2	May result in reduced contraceptive efficacy.
troglitazone	2	3	2	May result in possible loss of contraception.
troleandomycin	2	3	1	May result in altered contraceptive effectiveness and risk of hepatotoxicity.
valdecoxib	0	3	2	May result in increased exposure of norethindrone and ethinyl estradiol.
voriconazole	2	3	2	May result in increased levels of voriconazole and of ethinyl estradiol and norethindrone.
warfarin	2	3	2	May result in decreased or increased anticoagulant effectiveness.
ETODOLAC				
acenocoumarol	2	3	2	May result in increased risk of bleeding.
ACE Inhibitors *(alacepril, benazepril, captopril, cilazapril, delapril, enalapril maleate, enalaprilat, fosinopril, imidapril, lisinopril, moexipril, pentopril,*	2	3	2	May result in decreased antihypertensive and natriuretic effects.

perindopril, quinapril, ramipril, spirapril, temocapril, trandolapril, zofenopril)				
clopidogrel	2	3	2	May result in increased risk of bleeding.
cyclosporine	2	3	2	May result in increased risk of cyclosporine toxicity (renal dysfunction, cholestasis, paresthesias).
danaparoid	1	2	2	May result in increased risk of bleeding and an increased risk of hematoma when neuraxial anesthesia is employed.
desvenlafaxine	0	2	2	May result in increased risk of bleeding.
dicumarol	2	3	2	May result in increased risk of bleeding.
ginkgo	2	2	2	May result in increased risk of bleeding.
LMWHs (ardeparin, certoparin, dalteparin, enoxaparin, nadroparin, parnaparin, reviparin, tinzaparin)	1	2	2	May result in increased risk of bleeding.
Loop Diuretics (azosemide, bumetanide, ethacrynic acid, furosemide, piretanide, torsemide)	2	3	2	May result in decreased diuretic and antihypertensive efficacy.
phenprocoumon	2	3	2	May result in increased risk of bleeding.
piretanide	2	3	2	May result in decreased diuretic and antihypertensive efficacy.

Potassium-Sparing Diuretics (*amiloride, canrenoate, eplerenone, spironolactone, triamterene, torsemide*)	2	3	2	May result in reduced diuretic effectiveness, hyperkalemia, or possible nephrotoxicity.
SSRIs (*citalopram, clovoxamine, femoxetine, fleinoxan, fluoxetine, nefazodone, paroxetine, sertraline, venlafaxine, zimeldine*)	0	3	2	May result in increased risk of bleeding.
Sulfonylureas (*acetohexamide, chlorpropamide, gliclazide, glimepiride, glipizide, gliquidone, glyburide, tolazamide, tolbutamide*)	2	3	2	May result in increased risk of hypoglycemia.
tacrolimus	2	2	2	May result in acute renal failure.
Thiazide Diuretics (*bemetizide, bendroflumethiazide, benzthiazide, buthiazide, chlorthiazide, chlorthalidone, clopamide, cyclopenthiazide, cyclothiazide, HCTZ, hydroflumethiazide, indapamide, methyclothiazide, metolazone, polythiazide, quinethazone, trichlormethiazide, xipamide*)	2	3	2	May result in decreased diuretic and antihypertensive efficacy.
venlafaxine	0	3	2	May result in increased risk of bleeding.

ETONOGESTREL

Drug	Onset	Severity		Effect
alprazolam	2	3	2	May result in increased risk of alprazolam toxicity (CNS depression, hypotension).
ampicillin	2	3	2	May result in decreased contraceptive effectiveness.
amprenavir	2	3	2	May result in decreased serum concentrations of amprenavir; loss of contraceptive efficacy.
aprepitant	2	3	2	May result in reduced efficacy of combination contraceptives.
bacampicillin	2	3	2	May result in decreased contraceptive effectiveness.
betamethasone	2	3	2	May result in increased corticosteroid effects.
bexarotene	2	3	2	May result in decreased contraceptive effectiveness.
bosentan	2	3	2	May result in decreased contraceptive effectiveness.
caffeine	1	3	2	May result in enhanced CNS stimulation.
carbamazepine	2	3	2	May result in decreased plasma concentrations of estrogens and in estrogen effectiveness.
cyclosporine	2	3	2	May result in increased risk of cyclosporine toxicity (renal dysfunction, cholestasis, paresthesias).
fosamprenavir	2	2	1	May result in decreased serum concentrations of amprenavir, altered hormonal levels, and an increased risk of hepatotoxicity.

ONSET: 0 - NOT SPECIFIED 1 - RAPID 2 - DELAYED   SEVERITY: 1 - CONTRAINDICATED 2 - MAJOR 3 - MODERATE

fosphenytoin	2	3	2	May result in decreased contraceptive effectiveness.
griseofulvin	2	3	1	May result in decreased contraceptive effectiveness.
lamotrigine	2	3	2	May result in altered (increased or decreased) plasma lamotrigine concentrations.
licorice	2	3	2	May result in increased risk of fluid retention and elevated blood pressure.
modafinil	2	3	2	May result in decreased contraceptive bioavailability and reduced contraceptive effectiveness.
mycophenolate mofetil	0	3	2	May result in decreased contraceptive exposure.
nelfinavir	2	3	2	May result in contraceptive failure.
nevirapine	2	3	2	May result in loss of contraceptive efficacy.
oxcarbazepine	2	3	2	May result in decreased contraceptive effectiveness.
phenobarbital	2	3	2	May result in decreased plasma concentrations of estrogens and in contraceptive effectiveness.
phenytoin	2	3	2	May result in decreased contraceptive effectiveness.
primidone	2	3	2	May result in decreased contraceptive effectiveness.
rifampin	2	3	1	May result in decreased plasma concentrations of estrogens and in contraceptive effectiveness.
rosuvastatin	0	3	2	May result in increased exposure to ethinyl estradiol and norgestrel.

St. John's wort	2	3	1	May result in decreased plasma concentrations of estrogens and in contraceptive effectiveness.
topiramate	2	3	2	May result in reduced contraceptive efficacy.
troglitazone	2	3	2	May result in possible loss of contraception.
troleandomycin	2	3	1	May result in altered contraceptive effectiveness and risk of hepatotoxicity.
warfarin	2	3	2	May result in decreased or increased anticoagulant effectiveness.
EZETIMIBE				
cholestyramine	0	3	1	May result in reduced ezetimibe plasma concentrations.
colesevelam	0	3	2	May result in reduced ezetimibe plasma concentrations.
colestipol	0	3	2	May result in reduced ezetimibe plasma concentrations.
cyclosporine	0	3	2	May result in increased ezetimibe and cyclosporine plasma concentrations.
fenofibrate	2	3	2	May result in increased ezetimibe concentrations and an increased risk of cholelithiasis.
gemfibrozil	2	2	2	May result in increased ezetimibe concentrations and an increased risk of cholelithiasis.
FAMOTIDINE				
atazanavir	0	2	2	May result in reduced atazanavir plasma concentrations.

ONSET: 0 = NOT SPECIFIED 1 = RAPID 2 = DELAYED   SEVERITY: 1 = CONTRAINDICATED 2 = MAJOR 3 = MODERATE

cefditoren pivoxil	2	3	2	May result in decreased cefditoren serum concentrations.
cefpodoxime proxetil	1	3	2	May result in decreased cefpodoxime effectiveness.
cyclosporine	2	3	2	May result in decreased cyclosporine concentrations.
itraconazole	2	3	1	May result in loss of itraconazole efficacy.
FELODIPINE				
amiodarone	1	2	2	May result in bradycardia, atrioventricular block and/or sinus arrest.
amprenavir	2	3	2	May result in increased plasma concentrations of felodipine.
β-Blockers (*acebutolol, alprenolol, atenolol, betaxolol, bevantolol, bisoprolol, bucindolol, carteolol, carvedilol, celiprolol, dilevalol, esmolol, labetalol, levobunolol, mepindolol, metipranolol, metoprolol, nadolol, nebivolol, oxprenolol, penbutolol, pindolol, propranolol, sotalol, talinolol, tertatolol, timolol*)	1	3	2	May result in hypotension and/or bradycardia.
cyclosporine	2	2	2	May result in increased risk of felodipine toxicity.
dalfopristin	2	3	2	May result in increased risk of felodipine toxicity (dizziness, hypotension, flushing, headache, peripheral edema).

fentanyl	1	2	2	May result in severe hypotension.
fluconazole	2	3	2	May result in increased felodipine serum concentrations and toxicity (dizziness, hypotension, flushing, headache, peripheral edema).
grapefruit juice	1	3	1	May result in severe hypotension, myocardial ischemia, increased vasodilator side effects.
indinavir	0	3	2	May result in increased plasma concentrations of CCB.
itraconazole	2	3	2	May result in increased felodipine serum concentrations and toxicity (dizziness, hypotension, flushing, headache, peripheral edema).
ketoconazole	2	3	2	May result in increased felodipine serum concentrations and toxicity (dizziness, hypotension, flushing, headache, peripheral edema).
magnesium	1	3	2	May result in hypotension.
mepindolol	1	3	2	May result in hypotension and/or bradycardia.
mibefradil	1	2	2	May result in severe bradycardia and hypotension.
nadolol	1	3	2	May result in hypotension and/or bradycardia.
nelfinavir	2	3	2	May result in increased plasma concentrations of felodipine.
oxcarbazepine	2	3	2	May result in decreased felodipine exposure.
phenobarbital	2	3	2	May result in decreased felodipine effectiveness.

ONSET: 0 - NOT SPECIFIED 1 - RAPID 2 - DELAYED   SEVERITY: 1 - CONTRAINDICATED 2 - MAJOR 3 - MODERATE

quinupristin	2	3	2	May result in increased risk of felodipine toxicity (dizziness, hypotension, flushing, headache, peripheral edema).
rifapentine	2	3	2	May result in decreased CCB effectiveness.
saquinavir	1	3	2	May result in increased risk of felodipine toxicity (dizziness, headache, flushing, peripheral edema, hypotension, cardiac arrhythmias).
St. John's wort	2	3	2	May result in reduced bioavailability of CCB.
voriconazole	0	3	2	May result in increased plasma concentrations of CCB.
FENOFIBRATE				
acenocoumarol	2	2	2	May result in increased INR and risk of bleeding events.
anisindione	2	2	2	May result in increased INR and risk of bleeding events.
atorvastatin	0	2	2	May result in increased risk of myopathy or rhabdomyolysis.
cerivastatin	2	2	2	May result in increased risk of myopathy or rhabdomyolysis.
colesevelam	1	3	2	May result in decreased fenofibrate bioavailability and reduced effectiveness.
colestipol	1	3	2	May result in decreased fenofibrate bioavailability and reduced effectiveness.
dicumarol	2	2	2	May result in increased INR and risk of bleeding events.

ezetimibe	2	3	2	May result in increased ezetimibe concentrations and an increased risk of cholelithiasis.
fluvastatin	0	2	2	May result in increased risk of myopathy or rhabdomyolysis.
lovastatin	0	2	2	May result in increased risk of myopathy or rhabdomyolysis.
phenindione	2	2	2	May result in increased INR and risk of bleeding events.
phenprocoumon	2	2	2	May result in increased INR and risk of bleeding events.
pravastatin	0	2	2	May result in increased risk of myopathy or rhabdomyolysis.
warfarin	2	2	2	May result in increased INR and risk of bleeding events.
FENTANYL				
amprenavir	2	3	1	May result in increased risk of fentanyl toxicity (CNS depression, respiratory depression).
atazanavir	2	3	1	May result in increased risk of fentanyl toxicity (CNS depression, respiratory depression).
azithromycin	2	3	2	May result in increased or prolonged opioid effects (CNS depression, respiratory depression).

ONSET: 0 - NOT SPECIFIED 1 - RAPID 2 - DELAYED   SEVERITY: 1 - CONTRAINDICATED 2 - MAJOR 3 - MODERATE

β-Blockers (*acebutolol, alprenolol, atenolol, betaxolol, bevantolol, bisoprolol, bucindolol, carteolol, carvedilol, celiprolol, dilevalol, esmolol, labetalol, levobunolol, mepindolol, metipranolol, metoprolol, nadolol, nebivolol, oxprenolol, penbutolol, pindolol, propranolol, sotalol, talinolol, tertatolol, timolol*)	1	2	2	May result in severe hypotension.
Barbiturates (*amobarbital, aprobarbital, butabarbital, butalbital, mephobarbital, methohexital, pentobarbital, phenobarbital, primidone, secobarbital, thiopental*)	0	2	2	May result in additive respiratory depression.
BZDs (*adinazolam, alprazolam, bromazepam, brotizolam, chlordiazepoxide, clobazam, clonazepam, clorazepate, diazepam, estazolam, flunitrazepam, flurazepam, halazepam, ketazolam, lorazepam, lormetazepam, lormetazepam, medazepam, midazolam, nitrazepam, nordazepam, oxazepam, prazepam, temazepam, triazolam*)	0	2	2	May result in additive respiratory depression.

CCBs (amlodipine, bepridil, diltiazem, felodipine, flunarizine, gallopamil, isradipine, lacidipine, lercanidipine, lidoflazine, manidipine, nicardipine, nifedipine, nilvadipine, nimodipine, nisoldipine, nitrendipine, prandipine, verapamil)	1	2	2	May result in severe hypotension.
carbamazepine	2	3	2	May result in decreased plasma concentrations of fentanyl.
clarithromycin	2	2	2	May result in increased or prolonged opioid effects (CNS depression, respiratory depression).
clotrimazole	2	3	2	May result in increased or prolonged opioid effects (CNS depression, respiratory depression).
dirithromycin	2	3	2	May result in increased or prolonged opioid effects (CNS depression, respiratory depression).
econazole	2	3	2	May result in increased or prolonged opioid effects (CNS depression, respiratory depression).
erythromycin	2	3	2	May result in increased or prolonged opioid effects (CNS depression, respiratory depression).
fluconazole	2	2	2	May result in increased or prolonged opioid effects (CNS depression, respiratory depression).
fosamprenavir	2	3	1	May result in increased risk of fentanyl toxicity (CNS depression, respiratory depression).

ONSET: 0 = NOT SPECIFIED, 1 = RAPID, 2 = DELAYED   SEVERITY: 1 = CONTRAINDICATED, 2 = MAJOR, 3 = MODERATE

indinavir	2	3	1	May result in increased risk of fentanyl toxicity (CNS depression, respiratory depression).
itraconazole	2	2	2	May result in increased or prolonged opioid effects (CNS depression, respiratory depression).
josamycin	2	3	2	May result in increased or prolonged opioid effects (CNS depression, respiratory depression).
ketoconazole	2	2	2	May result in increased or prolonged opioid effects (CNS depression, respiratory depression).
lopinavir	2	3	1	May result in increased risk of fentanyl toxicity (CNS depression, respiratory depression).
mepartricin	2	3	2	May result in increased or prolonged opioid effects (CNS depression, respiratory depression).
miconazole	2	3	2	May result in increased or prolonged opioid effects (CNS depression, respiratory depression).
miokamycin	2	3	2	May result in increased or prolonged opioid effects (CNS depression, respiratory depression).
Muscle Relaxants, Centrally Acting (*carisoprodol, chlorzoxazone, dantrolene, mephenesin, meprobamate, metaxalone, methocarbamol*)	0	2	2	May result in additive respiratory depression.
naltrexone	1	1	2	May result in precipitation of opioid withdrawal symptoms; decreased opioid effectiveness.

nefazodone	2	2	2	May result in increased or prolonged opioid effects (CNS depression, respiratory depression).
nelfinavir	2	2	1	May result in increased risk of fentanyl toxicity (CNS depression, respiratory depression).
nevirapine	0	3	2	May result in decreased plasma concentrations of fentanyl.
Opioid Agonists/Antagonists (*buprenorphine, butorphanol, dezocine, nalbuphine, pentazocine*)	2	2	2	May result in precipitation of withdrawal symptoms (abdominal cramps, nausea, vomiting, lacrimation, rhinorrhea, anxiety, restlessness, elevation of temperature or piloerection).
phenytoin	2	3	2	May result in decreased plasma concentrations of fentanyl.
rifampin	2	3	2	May result in decreased plasma concentrations of fentanyl and potentially reduced analgesic effect.
ritonavir	2	2	1	May result in increased risk of fentanyl toxicity (CNS depression, respiratory depression).
rokitamycin	2	3	2	May result in increased or prolonged opioid effects (CNS depression, respiratory depression).
roxithromycin	2	3	2	May result in increased or prolonged opioid effects (CNS depression, respiratory depression).
saquinavir	2	3	1	May result in increased risk of fentanyl toxicity (CNS depression, respiratory depression).

ONSET: 0 = NOT SPECIFIED 1 = RAPID 2 = DELAYED   SEVERITY: 1 = CONTRAINDICATED 2 = MAJOR 3 = MODERATE

sibutramine	1	2	2	May result in increased risk of serotonin syndrome (hypertension, hypothermia, myoclonus, mental status changes).
spiramycin	2	3	2	May result in increased or prolonged opioid effects (CNS depression, respiratory depression).
tranylcypromine	1	2	2	May result in cardiac instability, hyperpyrexia, coma, and severe and unpredictable potentiation of opioid analgesic effects.
troleandomycin	2	2	2	May result in increased or prolonged opioid effects (CNS depression, respiratory depression).
FEXOFENADINE				
Antacids (*aluminum carbonate, basic, aluminum hydroxide, aluminum phosphate, dihydroxyaluminum aminoacetate, dihydroxyaluminum sodium carbonate, magaldrate, magnesium carbonate, magnesium hydroxide, magnesium oxide, magnesium trisilicate*)	1	3	2	May result in decreased fexofenadine efficacy.
apple juice	1	3	2	May result in reduced effectiveness of fexofenadine.
grapefruit juice	1	3	1	May result in reduced effectiveness of fexofenadine.
orange juice	1	3	2	May result in reduced fexofenadine exposure.

FINASTERIDE

FLUCONAZOLE

acenocoumarol	2	2	2	May result in increased risk of bleeding.
alfentanil	1	3	2	May result in prolonged alfentanil effects.
amitriptyline	2	2	2	May result in increased risk of amitriptyline toxicity and an increased risk of cardiotoxicity (QT prolongation, torsades de pointes, cardiac arrest).
amlodipine	2	3	2	May result in increased amlodipine serum concentrations and toxicity (dizziness, hypotension, flushing, headache, peripheral edema).
astemizole	2	1	2	May result in cardiotoxicity (QT prolongation, torsades de pointes, cardiac arrest).
atevirdine	2	3	2	May result in increased atevirdine plasma concentrations.
carbamazepine	1	3	2	May result in increased risk of carbamazepine toxicity (ataxia, nystagmus, diplopia, headache, vomiting, apnea, seizures, coma).
celecoxib	2	3	2	May result in increased celecoxib plasma concentrations.
cerivastatin	2	2	2	May result in increased risk of myopathy or rhabdomyolysis.

ONSET: 0 - NOT SPECIFIED 1 - RAPID 2 - DELAYED   SEVERITY: 1 - CONTRAINDICATED 2 - MAJOR 3 - MODERATE

cimetidine	2	3	2	May result in decreased fluconazole effectiveness.
cisapride	2	1	2	May result in cardiotoxicity (QT prolongation, torsades de pointes, cardiac arrest).
clarithromycin	0	2	2	May result in increased risk of cardiotoxicity (QT prolongation, torsades de pointes, cardiac arrest).
cyclosporine	2	3	2	May result in increased risk of cyclosporine toxicity (renal dysfunction, cholestasis, paresthesias).
dicumarol	2	2	2	May result in increased risk of bleeding.
eplerenone	0	2	2	May result in increased eplerenone plasma concentrations and increased risk of eplerenone side effects.
Ergot Derivatives (*dihydroergotamine, ergoloid mesylates, ergonovine, ergotamine, methylergonovine*)	1	1	2	May result in increased risk of ergotism (nausea, vomiting, vasospastic ischemia).
felodipine	2	3	2	May result in increased felodipine serum concentrations and toxicity (dizziness, hypotension, flushing, headache, peripheral edema).
fentanyl	2	2	2	May result in increased or prolonged opioid effects (CNS depression, respiratory depression).
fosphenytoin	2	3	1	May result in increased risk of phenytoin toxicity (ataxia, hyperreflexia, nystagmus, tremors).
gemifloxacin	0	2	2	May result in increased risk of cardiotoxicity (QT prolongation, torsades de pointes, cardiac arrest).

glimepiride	1	3	1	May result in increased blood concentrations of glimepiride and an increased risk of hypoglycemia.
isradipine	2	2	2	May result in increased isradipine serum concentrations and toxicity (dizziness, hypotension, flushing, headache, peripheral edema) and an increased risk of cardiotoxicity (QT prolongation, torsades de pointes, cardiac arrest).
levofloxacin	2	2	2	May result in increased risk of QTc prolongation and torsades de pointes.
losartan	1	3	2	May result in decreased conversion of losartan to its active metabolite, E-3174.
methadone	0	3	2	May result in increased plasma methadone levels.
methysergide	1	1	2	May result in increased risk of ergotism (nausea, vomiting, vasospastic ischemia).
midazolam	1	3	1	May result in increased midazolam concentrations and potential midazolam toxicity (excessive sedation and prolonged hypnotic effects).
nevirapine	1	2	2	May result in increased nevirapine exposure.
nicardipine	2	3	2	May result in increased nicardipine serum concentrations and toxicity (dizziness, hypotension, flushing, headache, peripheral edema).

ONSET: 0 = NOT SPECIFIED 1 = RAPID 2 = DELAYED   SEVERITY: 1 = CONTRAINDICATED 2 = MAJOR 3 = MODERATE
EVIDENCE: 1 = EXCELLENT 2 = GOOD

INTERACTING DRUG	ONSET	SEVERITY	EVIDENCE	WARNING
nifedipine	2	3	2	May result in increased nifedipine serum concentrations and toxicity (dizziness, hypotension, flushing, headache, peripheral edema).
nitrofurantoin	2	2	2	May result in increased risk of hepatic and pulmonary toxicity.
nortriptyline	0	2	2	May result in increased risk of nortriptyline toxicity and an increased risk of cardiotoxicity (QT prolongation, torsades de pointes, cardiac arrest).
phenprocoumon	2	2	2	May result in increased risk of bleeding.
phenytoin	2	3	2	May result in increased risk of phenytoin toxicity (ataxia, hyperreflexia, nystagmus, tremors).
prednisone	2	3	2	May result in decreased metabolic degradation of prednisone and increased prednisone efficacy.
quetiapine	2	2	2	May result in increased quetiapine serum concentrations; an increased risk of cardiotoxicity (QT prolongation, torsades de pointes, cardiac arrest).
ramelteon	2	3	2	May result in increased exposure to ramelteon with increased risk of side effects.
rifabutin	2	2	1	May result in increased rifabutin serum concentrations and potential rifabutin toxicity (uveitis, ocular pain, photophobia, visual disturbances, loss of vision).

rifampin	2	3	1	May result in decreased fluconazole serum concentrations and antifungal activity.
rifapentine	2	3	2	May result in loss of fluconazole efficacy.
rosuvastatin	2	3	2	May result in increased rosuvastatin exposure and an increased risk of myopathy or rhabdomyolysis.
simvastatin	2	2	2	May result in increased risk of myopathy or rhabdomyolysis.
sirolimus	2	2	2	May result in increased risk of sirolimus toxicity (anemia, leukopenia, thrombocytopenia, hypokalemia, diarrhea).
tacrolimus	1	3	1	May result in increased tacrolimus concentration.
terfenadine	1	1	2	May result in increased serum concentrations of terfenadine and its active metabolite, and an increased risk of cardiotoxicity (QT prolongation, torsades de pointes, cardiac arrest).
tipranavir	0	3	1	May result in increased exposure to tipranavir with increased risk of side effects.
tretinoin	1	3	2	May result in increased risk of tretinoin toxicity.
triazolam	1	2	1	May result in increased triazolam concentrations and potential triazolam toxicity (excessive sedation and prolonged hypnotic effects).

ONSET: 0 - NOT SPECIFIED, 1 - RAPID, 2 - DELAYED   SEVERITY: 1 - CONTRAINDICATED, 2 - MAJOR, 3 - MODERATE

trimetrexate	2	3	2	May result in increased trimetrexate toxicity (bone marrow suppression, renal & hepatic dysfunction, and gastrointestinal ulceration).
valdecoxib	0	3	2	May result in increased valdecoxib plasma exposure and, potentially, valdecoxib adverse effects (headache, nausea, vomiting, abdominal pain).
warfarin	2	3	2	May result in increased risk of bleeding.
FLUOXETINE				
alprazolam	1	3	2	May result in increased risk of alprazolam toxicity (somnolence, dizziness, ataxia, slurred speech, hypotension, psychomotor impairment).
Anticoagulants (*abciximab, acenocoumarol, ancrod, anisindione, antithrombin III human, bivalirudin, cilostazol, clopidogrel, danaparoid, defibrotide, dermatan sulfate, dicumarol, eptifibatide, fondaparinux, lamifiban, pentosan polysulfate sodium, phenindione, phenprocoumon, sibrafiban, warfarin, xemilofiban*)	0	2	2	May result in an increased risk of bleeding.
Antiplatelet Agents (*abciximab, anagrelide, aspirin, cilostazol, clopidogrel, dipyridamole, epoprostenol, eptifibatide, iloprost,*	0	2	2	May result in an increased risk of bleeding.

lamifiban, lexipafant, sulfinpyrazone, sulodexide, ticlopidine, tirofiban, xemilofiban)				
bupropion	2	3	2	May result in increased plasma levels of fluoxetine.
buspirone	2	3	2	May result in worsening of psychiatric symptoms.
carbamazepine	2	3	2	May result in carbamazepine toxicity (ataxia, nystagmus, diplopia, headache, vomiting, apnea, seizures, coma).
clarithromycin	2	2	2	May result in delirium and psychosis.
clozapine	2	3	2	May result in increased risk of clozapine toxicity (sedation, seizures, hypotension).
cyclobenzaprine	2	3	2	May result in increased risk of QT prolongation.
cyproheptadine	1	3	2	May result in decreased fluoxetine efficacy.
delavirdine	2	3	2	May result in increased trough delavirdine concentrations.
digoxin	2	3	2	May result in increased risk of digoxin toxicity (nausea, vomiting, arrhythmias).
duloxetine	0	3	2	May result in increased duloxetine and fluoxetine serum concentrations and risk of adverse effects.
eletriptan	2	2	2	May result in increased risk of serotonin syndrome.

ONSET: 0 - NOT SPECIFIED 1 - RAPID 2 - DELAYED   SEVERITY: 1 - CONTRAINDICATED 2 - MAJOR 3 - MODERATE

Drug			Effect
Ergot Derivatives (*dihydroergotamine, ergoloid mesylates, ergonovine, ergotamine, methylergonovine, methysergide*)	0	1	2	May result in increased risk of ergotism (nausea, vomiting, vasospastic ischemia).
fluphenazine	2	3	2	May result in increased risk of developing acute parkinsonism.
fosphenytoin	2	3	1	May result in increased risk of phenytoin toxicity (ataxia, hyperreflexia, nystagmus, tremor).
frovatriptan	2	2	2	May result in increased risk of serotonin syndrome.
galantamine	0	3	2	May result in increased galantamine plasma concentrations.
gemifloxacin	0	2	2	May result in increased risk of cardiotoxicity (QT prolongation, torsades de pointes, cardiac arrest).
ginkgo	2	3	2	May result in increased risk of serotonin syndrome (hypertension, hyperthermia, myoclonus, mental status changes).
haloperidol	2	2	2	May result in haloperidol toxicity (pseudoparkinsonism, akathisia, tongue stiffness) and an increased risk of cardiotoxicity (QT prolongation, torsades de pointes, cardiac arrest).

iproniazid	1	1	2	May result in CNS toxicity or serotonin syndrome (hypertension, hyperthermia, myoclonus, mental status changes).
lithium	2	3	1	May result in possible increased lithium concentrations and/or an increased risk of SSRI-related serotonin syndrome (hypertension, hyperthermia, myoclonus, mental status changes).
metoprolol	2	3	2	May result in increased risk of metoprolol adverse effects (shortness of breath, bradycardia, hypotension, acute heart failure).
moclobemide	1	1	2	May result in CNS toxicity or serotonin syndrome (hypertension, hyperthermia, myoclonus, mental status changes).
naratriptan	2	2	2	May result in increased risk of serotonin syndrome.
nialamide	1	1	2	May result in CNS toxicity or serotonin syndrome (hypertension, hyperthermia, myoclonus, mental status changes).

NSAIDs (aceclofenac, acemetacin, alclofenac, apazone, aspirin, benoxaprofen, bromfenac, bufexamac, carprofen, celecoxib, clometacin, clonixin, dexketoprofen, diclofenac, diflunisal, dipyrone, dofetilide, droxicam, etodolac, etofenamate, felbinac, fenbufen, fenoprofen, fentiazac, floctafenine, flufenamic acid, flurbiprofen, ibuprofen, indomethacin, indoprofen, isoxicam, ketoprofen, ketorolac, lornoxicam, meclofenamate, mefenamic acid, meloxicam, nabumetone, naproxen, niflumic acid, nimesulide, oxaprozin, oxyphenbutazone, phenylbutazone, pirazolac, piroxicam, pirprofen, propyphenazon, proquazone, rofecoxib, sulindac, suprofen, tenidap, tenoxicam, tiaprofenic acid, ticrynafen, tolmetin, zomepirac)	0	3	2	May result in increased risk of bleeding.
pargyline	1	1	2	May result in CNS toxicity or serotonin syndrome (hypertension, hyperthermia, myoclonus, mental status changes).
paroxetine	2	3	2	May result in fluoxetine toxicity (dry mouth, sedation, urinary retention).

Drug	Onset		Severity	Description
pentazocine	1	3	2	May result in hypertension, diaphoresis, ataxia, flushing, nausea, dizziness, and anxiety.
phenytoin	2	3	2	May result in increased risk of phenytoin toxicity (ataxia, hyperreflexia, nystagmus, tremor).
pimozide	0	1	2	May result in bradycardia, somnolence, and potentially increased risk of cardiotoxicity (QT prolongation, torsades de pointes, cardiac arrest).
procarbazine	1	1	1	May result in CNS toxicity or serotonin syndrome (hypertension, hyperthermia, myoclonus, mental status changes).
propafenone	1	2	2	May result in increased serum propafenone concentrations and an increased risk of cardiotoxicity (QT prolongation, torsades de pointes, cardiac arrest).
rasagiline	0	2	2	May result in CNS toxicity or serotonin syndrome (hypertension, hyperthermia, myoclonus, mental status changes).
risperidone	0	3	2	May result in increased risk of risperidone adverse effects such as serotonin syndrome (hypertension, hyperthermia, myoclonus, mental status changes), extrapyramidal effects, and cardiotoxicity (QT prolongation, torsades de pointes, cardiac arrest) due to increased plasma risperidone levels.
ritonavir	2	3	1	May result in alterations in cardiac and/or neurologic function.

ONSET: 0 - NOT SPECIFIED 1 - RAPID 2 - DELAYED   SEVERITY: 1 - CONTRAINDICATED 2 - MAJOR 3 - MODERATE

rizatriptan	2	2	2	May result in increased risk of serotonin syndrome.
sibutramine	1	2	2	May result in increased risk of serotonin syndrome (hypertension, hyperthermia, myoclonus, mental status changes).
St. John's wort	1	2	2	May result in increased risk of serotonin syndrome (hypertension, hyperthermia, myoclonus, mental status changes).
TCAs (amitriptyline, amoxapine, clomipramine, desipramine, dibenzepin, dothiepin, doxepin, imipramine, lofepramine, melitracen, nortriptyline, trimipramine)	0	2	2	May result in tricyclic antidepressant toxicity (dry mouth, urinary retention, sedation) and increased risk of cardiotoxicity (QT prolongation, torsades de pointes, cardiac arrest).
terfenadine	2	1	2	May result in cardiotoxicity (QT prolongation, torsades de pointes, cardiac arrest).
thioridazine	1	1	2	May result in increased risk of cardiotoxicity (QT prolongation, torsades de pointes, cardiac arrest).
toloxatone	1	1	2	May result in CNS toxicity or serotonin syndrome (hypertension, hyperthermia, myoclonus, mental status changes).
tramadol	1	2	2	May result in increased risk of seizures and serotonin syndrome (hypertension, hyperthermia, myoclonus, mental status changes); increased concentrations of tramadol and decreased concentrations of tramadol active metabolite, M1.

tranylcypromine	1	1	2	May result in CNS toxicity or serotonin syndrome (hypertension, hyperthermia, myoclonus, mental status changes).
trazodone	2	2	2	May result in trazodone toxicity (sedation, dry mouth, urinary retention) or serotonin syndrome (hypertension, hyperthermia, myoclonus, mental status changes).
tryptophan	2	2	2	May result in serotonin syndrome (hypertension, hyperthermia, myoclonus, mental status changes).
warfarin	2	3	2	May result in increased risk of bleeding.
FLUTICASONE				
darunavir	0	2	2	May result in increased fluticasone plasma concentrations.
ritonavir	2	2	1	May result in increased plasma fluticasone exposure and decreased plasma cortisol, the latter which may increase risk of developing Cushing's syndrome.
tipranavir	0	2	2	May result in increased plasma fluticasone levels and decreased plasma cortisol concentrations.
FOLIC ACID				
phenytoin	2	3	2	May result in decreased phenytoin effectiveness.
FOSINOPRIL				
aliskiren	0	3	2	May result in hyperkalemia.

ONSET: 0 – NOT SPECIFIED 1 – RAPID 2 – DELAYED   SEVERITY: 1 – CONTRAINDICATED 2 – MAJOR 3 – MODERATE

bupivacaine	2	3	2	May result in bradycardia and hypotension with loss of consciousness.
capsaicin	1	3	2	May result in increased risk of cough.
digoxin measurement	0	3	2	May result in false decreases in serum digoxin level due to unknown mechanism.
lithium	2	3	2	May result in lithium toxicity (weakness, tremor, excessive thirst, confusion) and/or nephrotoxicity.
Loop Diuretics (azosemide, bumetanide, ethacrynic acid, furosemide, piretanide, torsemide)	1	3	2	May result in postural hypotension (first dose).
nesiritide	2	3	2	May result in increased symptomatic hypotension.
NSAIDs (aceclofenac, acemetacin, alclofenac, apazone, aspirin, benoxaprofen, bromfenac, bufexamac, carprofen, celecoxib, clometacin, clonixin, dexketoprofen, diclofenac, diflunisal, dipyrone, dofetilide, droxicam, etodolac, etofenamate, felbinac, fenbufen, fenoprofen, fentiazac, floctafenine, flufenamic acid, flurbiprofen, ibuprofen, indomethacin, indoprofen, isoxicam, ketoprofen, ketorolac, lornoxicam, meclofenamate,	2	3	2	May result in decreased antihypertensive and natriuretic effects.

mefanamic acid, meloxicam, nabumetone, naproxen, niflumic acid, nimesulide, oxaprozin, oxyphenbutazone, phenylbutazone, pirazolac, piroxicam, pirprofen, propyphenazon, proquazone, rofecoxib, sulindac, suprofen, tenidap, tenoxicam, tiaprofenic acid, ticrynafen, tolmetin, zomepirac)				
potassium	2	2	2	May result in hyperkalemia.
Potassium-Sparing Diuretics (amiloride, canrenoate, eplerenone, spironolactone, triamterene, torsemide)	2	2	2	May result in hyperkalemia.
Thiazide Diuretics (bemetizide, bendroflumethiazide, benzthiazide, buthiazide, chlorthiazide, chlorthalidone, clopamide, cyclopenthiazide, cyclothiazide, HCTZ, hydroflumethiazide, indapamide, methyclothiazide, metolazone, polythiazide, quinethazone, trichlormethiazide, xipamide)	1	3	2	May result in postural hypotension (first dose).

FUROSEMIDE

Drug				Effect
ACE Inhibitors (*benazepril, cilazapril, delapril, fosinopril, lisinopril, pentopril, perindopril, spirapril, temocapril, trandolapril, zofenopril*)	1	3	2	May result in postural hypotension (first dose).
aliskiren	0	3	2	May result in decreased furosemide exposure and maximum plasma concentrations.
aspirin	1	3	2	May result in blunting of the diuretic effect of furosemide.
bepridil	2	2	2	May result in hypokalemia and subsequent cardiotoxicity (torsades de pointes).
cephaloridine	2	3	1	May result in increased risk of cephaloridine toxicity.
cholestyramine	1	3	2	May result in decreased furosemide effectiveness.
clofibrate	2	3	2	May result in muscle pain and stiffness, accentuation of diuretic effects, and elevations in serum transaminases and creatine phosphokinase.
colestipol	1	3	2	May result in decreased furosemide effectiveness.
dibekacin	1	3	2	May result in ototoxicity and/or nephrotoxicity.
digitoxin	2	2	2	May result in digitoxin toxicity (nausea, vomiting, cardiac arrhythmias).

digoxin	2	3	2	May result in digoxin toxicity (nausea, vomiting, cardiac arrhythmias).
dofetilide	0	2	2	May result in increased risk of cardiotoxicity (QT prolongation, torsades de pointes, cardiac arrest).
food	1	3	1	May result in decreased furosemide exposure and efficacy.
gentamicin	1	3	2	May result in ototoxicity and/or nephrotoxicity and altered plasma levels of gentamicin.
germanium	2	3	2	May result in increased risk of diuretic resistance.
ginseng	2	3	2	May result in increased risk of diuretic resistance.
gossypol	2	3	2	May result in increased risk of hypokalemia.
licorice	2	3	2	May result in increased risk of hypokalemia and/or reduced effectiveness of the diuretic.
lithium	2	2	2	May result in increased lithium concentrations and lithium toxicity (weakness, tremor, excessive thirst, confusion).
neomycin	1	3	2	May result in ototoxicity and/or nephrotoxicity.

ONSET: 0 - NOT SPECIFIED 1 - RAPID 2 - DELAYED   SEVERITY: 1 - CONTRAINDICATED 2 - MAJOR 3 - MODERATE

Drug				Effect
NSAIDs (aceclofenac, acemetacin, alclofenac, apazone, benoxaprofen, bromfenac, bufexamac, carprofen, celecoxib, clometacin, clonixin, dexketoprofen, diclofenac, diflunisal, dipyrone, dofetilide, droxicam, etodolac, etofenamate, felbinac, fenbufen, fenoprofen, fentiazac, floctafenine, flufenamic acid, flurbiprofen, ibuprofen, indomethacin, indoprofen, isoxicam, ketoprofen, ketorolac, lornoxicam, meclofenamate, mefenamic acid, meloxicam, nabumetone, naproxen, niflumic acid, nimesulide, oxaprozin, oxyphenbutazone, phenylbutazone, pirazolac, piroxicam, pirprofen, propyphenazon, proquazone, rofecoxib, sulindac, suprofen, tenidap, tenoxicam, tiaprofenic acid, ticrynafen, tolmetin, zomepirac)	2	3	2	May result in decreased diuretic and antihypertensive efficacy.
pancuronium	1	3	2	May result in increased or decreased neuromuscular blockade.
sotalol	0	2	2	May result in increased risk of cardiotoxicity (QT prolongation, torsades de pointes, cardiac arrest).
tobramycin	1	3	2	May result in ototoxicity and/or nephrotoxicity.

tubocurarine	1	3	2	May result in prolongation of neuromuscular blockade.
vecuronium	1	3	2	May result in increased or decreased neuromuscular blockade.

GABAPENTIN

Antacids (aluminum carbonate, basic, aluminum hydroxide, aluminum phosphate, dihydroxyaluminum aminoacetate, dihydroxyaluminum sodium carbonate, fludrocortisone, fluocortolone, hydrocortisone, magaldrate, magnesium carbonate, magnesium hydroxide, magnesium oxide, magnesium trisilicate)	1	3	2	May result in decreased gabapentin effectiveness.
ginkgo	2	3	2	May result in decreased anticonvulsant effectiveness.
urine total protein measurement	0	3	2	May result in false-positive urine protein measurement using Ames N-Multistix SG(R) dipstick test due to unknown mechanism.

GEMFIBROZIL

atorvastatin	2	2	1	May result in increased atorvastatin levels and an increased risk of myopathy or rhabdomyolysis.
bexarotene	2	3	2	May result in increased plasma concentrations of bexarotene.

cerivastatin	2	2	2	May result in increased risk of myopathy or rhabdomyolysis.
dicumarol	2	3	2	May result in increased risk of bleeding.
ezetimibe	2	2	2	May result in increased ezetimibe concentrations and an increased risk of cholelithiasis.
fluvastatin	2	2	2	May result in increased risk of myopathy or rhabdomyolysis.
glyburide	2	3	2	May result in hypoglycemia.
loperamide	2	3	1	May result in increased loperamide plasma concentration.
lovastatin	2	2	1	May result in increased risk of myopathy or rhabdomyolysis.
pioglitazone	1	3	1	May result in increased pioglitazone concentrations and potentially an increase risk of hypoglycemia.
pravastatin	2	2	2	May result in increased risk of myopathy or rhabdomyolysis.
repaglinide	1	1	2	May result in increased plasma concentrations of repaglinide.
rosiglitazone	1	3	2	May result in increased plasma concentrations of rosiglitazone.
simvastatin	2	2	2	May result in increased risk of myopathy or rhabdomyolysis.
warfarin	2	3	2	May result in increased risk of bleeding.

GLIMEPIRIDE

Drug				Effect
β-Blockers (*acebutolol, alprenolol, atenolol, betaxolol, bevantolol, bisoprolol, bucindolol, carteolol, carvedilol, celiprolol, dilevalol, esmolol, labetalol, levobunolol, mepindolol, metipranolol, metoprolol, nadolol, nebivolol, oxprenolol, penbutolol, pindolol, propranolol, sotalol, talinolol, tertatolol, timolol*)	2	3	2	May result in hypoglycemia, hyperglycemia, or hypertension.
bitter melon	1	3	2	May result in increased risk of hypoglycemia.
clorgyline	1	3	2	May result in excessive hypoglycemia, CNS depression, and seizures.
fenugreek	1	3	2	May result in increased risk of hypoglycemia.
FLQs (*alatrofloxacin, balofloxacin, cinoxacin, ciprofloxacin, clinafloxacin, enoxacin, fleroxacin, flumequine, gemifloxacin, grepafloxacin, levofloxacin, lomefloxacin, moxifloxacin, norfloxacin, ofloxacin, pefloxacin, prulifloxacin, rosoxacin, rufloxacin, sparfloxacin, temafloxacin, tosufloxacin, trovafloxacin*)	1	2	1	May result in changes in blood glucose and increased risk of hypoglycemia or hyperglycemia.

ONSET: 0 - NOT SPECIFIED, 1 - RAPID, 2 - DELAYED   SEVERITY: 1 - CONTRAINDICATED, 2 - MAJOR, 3 - MODERATE

fluconazole	1	3	1	May result in increased blood concentrations of glimepiride and an increased risk of hypoglycemia.
glucomannan	1	3	2	May result in increased risk of hypoglycemia.
guar gum	1	3	2	May result in increased risk of hypoglycemia.
NSAIDs (aceclofenac, acemetacin, alclofenac, apazone, benoxaprofen, bromfenac, bufexamac, carprofen, celecoxib, clometacin, clonixin, dexketoprofen, diclofenac, diflunisal, dipyrone, dofetilide, droxicam, etodolac, etofenamate, felbinac, fenbufen, fenoprofen, fentiazac, floctafenine, flufenamic acid, flurbiprofen, ibuprofen, indomethacin, indoprofen, isoxicam, ketoprofen, ketorolac, lornoxicam, meclofenamate, mefanamic acid, meloxicam, nabumetone, naproxen, niflumic acid, nimesulide, oxaprozin, oxyphenbutazone, phenylbutazone, pirazolac, piroxicam, pirprofen, propyphenazon, proquazone, rofecoxib, sulindac, suprofen, tenidap, tenoxicam, tiaprofenic acid, ticrynafen, tolmetin, zomepirac)	2	3	2	May result in increased risk of hypoglycemia.

psyllium	1	3	2	May result in increased risk of hypoglycemia.
St. John's wort	1	3	2	May result in hypoglycemia.
GLIPIZIDE				
β-Blockers (*acebutolol, alprenolol, atenolol, betaxolol, bevantolol, bisoprolol, bucindolol, carteolol, carvedilol, celiprolol, dilevalol, esmolol, labetalol, levobunolol, mepindolol, metipranolol, metoprolol, nadolol, nebivolol, oxprenolol, penbutolol, pindolol, propranolol, sotalol, talinolol, tertatolol, timolol*)	2	3	2	May result in hypoglycemia, hyperglycemia, or hypertension.
bitter melon	1	3	2	May result in increased risk of hypoglycemia.
cimetidine	2	3	2	May result in hypoglycemia.
cyclosporine	2	3	2	May result in increased risk of cyclosporine toxicity (renal dysfunction, cholestasis, paresthesias).
diazoxide	1	3	2	May result in decreased glipizide effectiveness.
fenugreek	1	3	2	May result in increased risk of hypoglycemia.

FLQs (*alatrofloxacin, balofloxacin, cinoxacin, ciprofloxacin, clinafloxacin, enoxacin, fleroxacin, flumequine, gemifloxacin, grepafloxacin, levofloxacin, lomefloxacin, moxifloxacin, norfloxacin, ofloxacin, pefloxacin, prulifloxacin, rosoxacin, rufloxacin, sparfloxacin, temafloxacin, tosufloxacin, trovafloxacin*)	1	2	1	May result in changes in blood glucose and increased risk of hypoglycemia or hyperglycemia.
glucomannan	1	3	2	May result in increased risk of hypoglycemia.
HCTZ	2	3	2	May result in decreased glipizide effectiveness.
MAOIs (*clorgyline, iproniazide, isocarboxazid, moclobemide, nialamide, pargyline, phenelzine, procarbazine, selegiline, toloxatone, tranylcypromine*).	1	3	2	May result in excessive hypoglycemia, CNS depression, and seizures.
NSAIDs (*aceclofenac, acemetacin, alclofenac, apazone, benoxaprofen, bromfenac, bufexamac, carprofen, celecoxib, clometacin, clonixin, dexketoprofen, diclofenac, diflunisal, dipyrone, dofetilide, droxicam, etodolac, etofenamate, felbinac, fenbufen, fenoprofen, fentiazac, floctafenine, flufenamic acid, flurbiprofen, ibuprofen, indomethacin, indoprofen, isoxicam,*	2	3	2	May result in increased risk of hypoglycemia.

ketoprofen, ketorolac, lornoxicam, meclofenamate, mefanamic acid, meloxicam, nabumetone, naproxen, niflumic acid, nimesulide, oxaprozin, oxyphenbutazone, phenylbutazone, pirazolac, piroxicam, pirprofen, propyphenazon, proquazone, rofecoxib, sulindac, suprofen, tenidap, tenoxicam, tiaprofenic acid, ticrynafen, tolmetin, zomepirac)				
psyllium	1	3	2	May result in increased risk of hypoglycemia.
ranitidine	2	3	2	May result in hypoglycemia.
St. John's wort	1	3	2	May result in hypoglycemia.
sulfadiazine	2	3	2	May result in enhanced hypoglycemic effects.
sulfamethoxazole	2	3	2	May result in enhanced hypoglycemic effects.
voriconazole	0	3	2	May result in increased plasma concentrations of sulfonylureas.
GLYBURIDE				
aspirin	2	3	2	May result in increased risk for hypoglycemia.

Drug/Substance				Effect
β-Blockers (*acebutolol, alprenolol, atenolol, betaxolol, bevantolol, bisoprolol, bucindolol, carteolol, carvedilol, celiprolol, dilevalol, esmolol, labetalol, levobunolol, mepindolol, metipranolol, metoprolol, nadolol, nebivolol, oxprenolol, penbutolol, pindolol, propranolol, sotalol, talinolol, tertatolol, timolol*)	2	3	2	May result in hypoglycemia, hyperglycemia, or hypertension.
bitter melon	1	3	2	May result in increased risk of hypoglycemia.
bosentan	1	1	2	May result in increased risk of liver enzyme elevations.
cyclosporine	2	3	2	May result in increased risk of cyclosporine toxicity (renal dysfunction, cholestasis, paresthesias).
ethanol	1	2	2	May result in prolonged hypoglycemia, disulfiram-like reactions.
fenugreek	1	3	2	May result in increased risk of hypoglycemia.
FLQs (*alatrofloxacin, balofloxacin, cinoxacin, ciprofloxacin, clinafloxacin, enoxacin, fleroxacin, flumequine, gemifloxacin, grepafloxacin, l evofloxacin, lomefloxacin, moxifloxacin, norfloxacin, ofloxacin, pefloxacin, prulifloxacin, rosoxacin, rufloxacin, sparfloxacin, temafloxacin, tosufloxacin, trovafloxacin*)	1	2	1	May result in changes in blood glucose and increased risk of hypoglycemia or hyperglycemia.

gemfibrozil	2	3	2	May result in hypoglycemia.
glucomannan	1	3	2	May result in increased risk of hypoglycemia.
MAOIs (clorgyline, iproniazid, isocarboxazid, moclobemide, nialamide, pargyline, phenelzine, procarbazine, selegiline, toloxatone, tranylcypromine)	1	3	2	May result in excessive hypoglycemia, CNS depression, and seizures.
NSAIDs (aceclofenac, acemetacin, alclofenac, apazone, benoxaprofen, bromfenac, bufexamac, carprofen, celecoxib, clometacin, clonixin, dexketoprofen, diclofenac, diflunisal, dipyrone, dofetilide, droxicam, etodolac, etofenamate, felbinac, fenbufen, fenoprofen, fentiazac, floctafenine, flufenamic acid, flurbiprofen, ibuprofen, indomethacin, indoprofen, isoxicam, ketoprofen, ketorolac, lornoxicam, meclofenamate, mefenamic acid, meloxicam, nabumetone, naproxen, niflumic acid, nimesulide, oxaprozin, oxyphenbutazone, phenylbutazone, pirazolac, piroxicam, pirprofen, propyphenazon, proquazone, rofecoxib, sulindac, suprofen, tenidap, tenoxicam, tiaprofenic acid, ticrynafen, tolmetin, zomepirac)	2	3	2	May result in increased risk of hypoglycemia.

ONSET: 0 = NOT SPECIFIED 1 = RAPID 2 = DELAYED   SEVERITY: 1 = CONTRAINDICATED 2 = MAJOR 3 = MODERATE

psyllium	1	3	2	May result in increased risk of hypoglycemia.
rifampin	2	3	2	May result in decreased glyburide effectiveness.
rifapentine	2	3	2	May result in decreased oral hypoglycemic effectiveness.
St. John's wort	1	3	2	May result in hypoglycemia.
sulfamethoxazole	2	3	2	May result in enhanced hypoglycemic effects.
voriconazole	0	3	2	May result in increased plasma concentrations of sulfonylureas.
warfarin	2	3	2	May result in increased risk of bleeding.

HYDROCHLOROTHIAZIDE

ACE Inhibitors (*alacepril, benazepril, captopril, cilazapril, delapril, enalapril maleate, enalaprilat, fosinopril, imidapril, lisinopril, moexipril, pentopril, perindopril, quinapril, ramipril, spirapril, temocapril, trandolapril, zofenopril*)	1	3	2	May result in postural hypotension (first dose).
acetaminophen measurement	1	3	2	May result in postural hypotension (first dose).
acetyldigoxin	1	3	2	May result in postural hypotension (first dose).
arsenic trioxide	1	3	2	May result in postural hypotension (first dose).
bepridil	1	3	2	May result in postural hypotension (first dose).
calcitriol	2	3	2	May result in hypercalcemia.

calcium carbonate	1	3	2	May result in postural hypotension (first dose).
carbamazepine	2	3	2	May result in hyponatremia.
chlorpropamide	1	3	2	May result in postural hypotension (first dose).
cholestyramine	1	3	2	May result in decreased HCTZ effectiveness.
colestipol	1	3	2	May result in postural hypotension (first dose).
cortisone	1	3	2	May result in postural hypotension (first dose).
cyclophosphamide	2	3	2	May result in hypercalcemia.
diazoxide	1	3	2	May result in postural hypotension (first dose).
dofetilide	1	3	2	May result in postural hypotension (first dose).
droperidol	1	3	2	May result in postural hypotension (first dose).
fludrocortisone	2	3	2	May result in the milk-alkali syndrome (hypercalcemia, metabolic alkalosis, renal failure).
fluorouracil	2	3	1	May result in decreased chlorpropamide effectiveness.
ginkgo	1	3	2	May result in postural hypotension (first dose).
glipizide	2	3	2	May result in decreased glipizide effectiveness.
glyburide	1	3	2	May result in postural hypotension (first dose).
gossypol	2	3	2	May result in increased risk of hypokalemia.
levomethadyl	2	3	2	May result in increased risk of hypokalemia.

ONSET: 0 = NOT SPECIFIED 1 = RAPID 2 = DELAYED   SEVERITY: 1 = CONTRAINDICATED 2 = MAJOR 3 = MODERATE
EVIDENCE: 1 = EXCELLENT 2 = GOOD

licorice	2	3	2	May result in increased risk of hypokalemia and/or reduced effectiveness of the diuretic.
lithium	2	2	2	May result in increased lithium concentrations and lithium toxicity (weakness, tremor, excessive thirst, confusion).
ma huang	2	3	2	May result in hypokalemia and subsequent cardiotoxicity (torsades de pointes).
memantine	2	3	2	May result in hyponatremia.
methotrexate	2	2	1	May result in digitalis toxicity (nausea, vomiting, arrhythmias).
methylprednisolone	2	2	1	May result in digitalis toxicity (nausea, vomiting, arrhythmias).
NSAIDs (aceclofenac, acemetacin, alclofenac, apazone, benoxaprofen, bromfenac, bufexamac, carprofen, celecoxib, clometacin, clonixin, dexketoprofen, diclofenac, diflunisal, dipyrone, dofetilide, droxicam, etodolac, etofenamate, felbinac, fenbufen, fenoprofen, fentiazac, floctafenine, flufenamic acid, flurbiprofen, ibuprofen, indomethacin, indoprofen, isoxicam, ketoprofen, ketorolac, lornoxicam, meclofenamate, mefanamic acid, meloxicam, nabumetone, naproxen, niflumic acid, nimesulide, oxaprozin, oxyphenbutazone, phenylbutazone,	1	3	2	May result in decreased HCTZ effectiveness.

pirazolac, piroxicam, pirprofen, propyphenazon, proquazone, rofecoxib, sulindac, suprofen, tenidap, tenoxicam, tiaprofenic acid, ticrynafen, tolmetin, zomepirac)				
ouabain	2	2	1	May result in digitalis toxicity (nausea, vomiting, arrhythmias).
porfimer	2	2	1	May result in digitalis toxicity (nausea, vomiting, arrhythmias).
prednisolone	2	2	1	May result in digitalis toxicity (nausea, vomiting, arrhythmias).
prednisone	2	2	1	May result in digitalis toxicity (nausea, vomiting, arrhythmias).
propranolol	0	1	2	May result in increased risk of cardiotoxicity (QT prolongation, torsades de pointes, cardiac arrhythmias).
sotalol	0	2	2	May result in increased risk of cardiotoxicity (QT prolongation, torsades de pointes, cardiac arrest).
topiramate	2	3	2	May result in increased topiramate exposure.
triamcinolone	2	3	2	May result in decreased glipizide effectiveness.
yohimbine	2	3	2	May result in myelosuppression (granulocytopenia).

ONSET: 0 - NOT SPECIFIED 1 - RAPID 2 - DELAYED   SEVERITY: 1 - CONTRAINDICATED 2 - MAJOR 3 - MODERATE

HYDROCODONE

Drug				Effect
Barbiturates (*amobarbital, aprobarbital, butabarbital, butalbital, mephobarbital, methohexital, pentobarbital, phenobarbital, secobarbital, thiopental*)	0	2	2	May result in additive respiratory depression.
BZDs (*adinazolam, alprazolam, bromazepam, brotizolam, chlordiazepoxide, clobazam, clonazepam, clorazepate, diazepam, estazolam, flunitrazepam, flurazepam, halazepam, ketazolam, lorazepam, lormetazepam, lormetazepam, medazepam, midazolam, nitrazepam, nordazepam, oxazepam, prazepam, temazepam, triazolam*)	0	2	2	May result in additive respiratory depression.
escitalopram	2	3	2	May result in increased risk of serotonin syndrome (tachycardia, hyperthermia, myoclonus, mental status changes).
Muscle Relaxants, Centrally Acting (*carisoprodol, chlorzoxazone, dantrolene, mephenesin, meprobamate, metaxalone, methocarbamol*)	0	2	2	May result in additive respiratory depression.
naltrexone	1	1	2	May result in precipitation of opioid withdrawal symptoms; decreased opioid effectiveness.

Opioid Agonists/Antagonists (buprenorphine, butorphanol, dezocine, nalbuphine, pentazocine)	2	2	2	May result in precipitation of withdrawal symptoms (abdominal cramps, nausea, vomiting, lacrimation, rhinorrhea, anxiety, restlessness, elevation of temperature or piloerection).
Opioid Analgesics (alfentanil, anileridine, codeine, fentanyl, hydrocodone, hydromorphone, levorphanol, meperidine, morphine, morphine sulfate liposome, oxycodone, oxymorphone, propoxyphene, remifentanil, sufentanil)	2	2	2	May result in precipitation of withdrawal symptoms (abdominal cramps, nausea, vomiting, lacrimation, rhinorrhea, anxiety, restlessness, elevation of temperature or piloerection).

HYDROXYCHLOROQUINE

digoxin	2	3	2	May result in increased serum digoxin concentrations.
metoprolol	2	3	2	May result in increased plasma levels of metoprolol.

IBANDRONATE SODIUM

food	1	3	2	May result in reduced ibandronate exposure.

IBUPROFEN

ACE Inhibitors (alacepril, benazepril, captopril, cilazapril, delapril, enalapril maleate, enalaprilat, fosinopril, imidapril, lisinopril, moexipril, pentopril, perindopril, quinapril, ramipril, spirapril, temocapril, trandolapril, zofenopril)	2	3	2	May result in decreased antihypertensive and natriuretic effects.
amikacin	0	3	2	May result in increased amikacin exposure.
aspirin	1	3	2	May result in decreased antiplatelet effect of aspirin.

ONSET: 0 - NOT SPECIFIED, 1 - RAPID, 2 - DELAYED   SEVERITY: 1 - CONTRAINDICATED, 2 - MAJOR, 3 - MODERATE

clopidogrel	2	3	2	May result in increased risk of bleeding.
cyclosporine	2	3	2	May result in increased risk of cyclosporine toxicity (renal dysfunction, cholestasis, paresthesias).
danaparoid	1	2	2	May result in increased risk of bleeding and an increased risk of hematoma when neuraxial anesthesia is employed.
desipramine	2	3	2	May result in increased risk of tricyclic toxicity (drowsiness, hypotension, akathisia).
desvenlafaxine	0	2	2	May result in increased risk of bleeding.
ginkgo	2	2	2	May result in increased risk of bleeding.
lithium	2	3	2	May result in increased risk of lithium toxicity (weakness, tremor, excessive thirst, confusion).
LMWHs (*ardeparin, certoparin, dalteparin, enoxaparin, nardroparin, parnaparin, reviparin, tinzaparin*)	1	2	2	May result in increased risk of bleeding.
Loop Diuretics (*azosemide, bumetanide, ethacrynic acid, furosemide, piretanide, torsemide*)	2	3	2	May result in decreased diuretic and antihypertensive efficacy.
methotrexate	2	2	2	May result in increased risk of methotrexate toxicity (leukopenia, thrombocytopenia, anemia, nephrotoxicity, mucosal ulcerations).
phenytoin	2	3	2	May result in increased risk of phenytoin toxicity (ataxia, hyperreflexia, nystagmus, tremor), especially in renally impaired patients.

Drug	Onset	Severity		Effect
Potassium-Sparing Diuretics (*amiloride, canrenoate, spironolactone, triamterene*)	2	3	2	May result in reduced diuretic effectiveness, hyperkalemia, or possible nephrotoxicity.
SSRIs (*citalopram, clovoxamine, femoxetine, fleseinoxan, fluoxetine, nefazodone, paroxetine, sertraline, venlafaxine, zimeldine*)	0	3	2	May result in increased risk of bleeding.
Sulfonylureas (*acetohexamide, chlorpropamide, gliclazide, glimepiride, glipizide, gliquidone, glyburide, tolazamide, tolbutamide*)	2	3	2	May result in increased risk of hypoglycemia.
tacrine	2	3	2	May result in symptoms of delirium (delusions, hallucinations, confusion, insomnia, tremor).
tacrolimus	2	2	2	May result in acute renal failure.
Thiazide Diuretics (*bemetizide, bendroflumethiazide, benthiazide, buthiazide, chlorothiazide, chlorthalidone, clopamide, cyclopenthiazide, cyclothiazide, HCTZ, hydroflumethiazide, indapamide, methyclothiazide, metolazone, polythiazide, quinethazone, trichlormethiazide, xipamide*)	2	3	2	May result in decreased diuretic and antihypertensive efficacy.
venlafaxine	0	3	2	May result in increased risk of bleeding.

ONSET: 0 - NOT SPECIFIED 1 - RAPID 2 - DELAYED   SEVERITY: 1 - CONTRAINDICATED 2 - MAJOR 3 - MODERATE

INSULIN

β-Blockers (*acebutolol, alprenolol, hypertension. atenolol, betaxolol, bevantolol, bisoprolol, bucindolol, carteolol, carvedilol, celiprolol, dilevalol, esmolol, labetalol, levobunolol, mepindolol, metipranolol, metoprolol, nadolol, nebivolol, oxprenolol, penbutolol, pindolol, propranolol, sotalol, talinolol, tertatolol, timolol*)	2	3	2	May result in hypoglycemia, hyperglycemia, or
bitter melon	1	3	2	May result in increased risk of hypoglycemia.
fenugreek	1	3	2	May result in increased risk of hypoglycemia.
FLQs (*alatrofloxacin, balofloxacin, cinoxacin, ciprofloxacin, clinafloxacin, enoxacin, fleroxacin, flumequine, gemifloxacin, grepafloxacin, levofloxacin, lomefloxacin, moxifloxacin, norfloxacin, ofloxacin, pefloxacin, prulifloxacin, rosoxacin, rufloxacin, sparfloxacin, temafloxacin, tosufloxacin, trovafloxacin*)	1	2	1	May result in changes in blood glucose and increased risk of hypoglycemia or hyperglycemia.

glucomannan	1	3	2	May result in increased risk of hypoglycemia.
guar gum	1	3	2	May result in increased risk of hypoglycemia.
MAOIs (*clorgyline, iproniazide, isocarboxazid, moclobemide, nialamide, pargyline, phenelzine, procarbazine, selegiline, toloxatone, tranylcypromine*)	1	3	2	May result in excessive hypoglycemia, CNS depression, and seizures.
psyllium	1	3	2	May result in increased risk of hypoglycemia.
St. John's wort	1	3	2	May result in hypoglycemia.
INSULIN LISPRO, RECOMBINANT				
β-Blockers (*acebutolol, alprenolol, atenolol, betaxolol, bevantolol, bisoprolol, bucindolol, carteolol, carvedilol, celiprolol, dilevalol, esmolol, labetalol, levobunolol, mepindolol, metipranolol, metoprolol, nadolol, nebivolol, oxprenolol, penbutolol, pindolol, propranolol, sotalol, talinolol, tertatolol, timolol*)	2	3	2	May result in hypoglycemia, hyperglycemia, or hypertension.
bitter melon	1	3	2	May result in increased risk of hypoglycemia.
fenugreek	1	3	2	May result in increased risk of hypoglycemia.

ONSET: 0 = NOT SPECIFIED 1 = RAPID 2 = DELAYED   SEVERITY: 1 = CONTRAINDICATED 2 = MAJOR 3 = MODERATE
EVIDENCE: 1 = EXCELLENT 2 = GOOD

FLQs (*alatrofloxacin, balofloxacin, ciprofloxacin, clinafloxacin, enoxacin, fleroxacin, flumequine, gatifloxacin, gemifloxacin, grepafloxacin, levofloxacin, lomefloxacin, moxifloxacin, norfloxacin, ofloxacin, pefloxacin, prulifloxacin, rufloxacin, sparfloxacin, temafloxacin, tosufloxacin, trovafloxacin mesylate*)	1	2	1	May result in changes in blood glucose and increased risk of hypoglycemia or hyperglycemia.
glucomannan	1	3	2	May result in increased risk of hypoglycemia.
guar gum	1	3	2	May result in increased risk of hypoglycemia.
MAOIs (*clorgyline, iproniazid, isocarboxazid, moclobemide, nialamide, pargyline, phenelzine, procarbazine, selegiline, toloxatone, tranylcypromine*)	1	3	2	May result in excessive hypoglycemia, CNS depression, and seizures.
psyllium	1	3	2	May result in increased risk of hypoglycemia.
St. John's wort	1	3	2	May result in hypoglycemia.
IPRATROPIUM				
betel nut	2	3	2	May result in reduced anticholinergic effect of ipratropium.
IRBESARTAN				
NSAIDs (*aceclofenac, acemetacin, alclofenac, apazone, aspirin, benoxaprofen, bromfenac, bufexamac,*	2	3	2	May result in decreased antihypertensive and natriuretic effects.

carprofen, celecoxib, clometacin,
clonixin, dexketoprofen, diclofenac,
diflunisal, dipyrone, dofetilide,
droxicam, etodolac, etofenamate,
felbinac, fenbufen, fenoprofen,
fentiazac, floctafenine, flufenamic acid,
flurbiprofen, ibuprofen, indomethacin,
indoprofen, isoxicam, ketoprofen,
ketorolac, lornoxicam, meclofenamate,
mefanamic acid, meloxicam,
nabumetone, naproxen, niflumic acid,
nimesulide, oxaprozin, oxyphenbutazone,
phenylbutazone, pirazolac, piroxicam,
pirprofen, propyphenazon, proquazone,
rofecoxib, sulindac, suprofen, tenidap,
tenoxicam, tiaprofenic acid, ticrynafen,
tolmetin, zomepirac)

IRON				
dairy food	1	3	2	May result in decreased iron bioavailability.
demeclocycline	2	3	2	May result in decreased demeclocycline and iron effectiveness.
doxycycline	2	3	2	May result in decreased tetracycline and iron effectiveness.

ONSET: 0 = NOT SPECIFIED, 1 = RAPID, 2 = DELAYED   SEVERITY: 1 = CONTRAINDICATED, 2 = MAJOR, 3 = MODERATE

gatifloxacin	1	3	2	May result in decreased gatifloxacin effectiveness.
grepafloxacin	1	3	2	May result in decreased efficacy of grepafloxacin.
levodopa	1	3	2	May result in decreased levodopa effectiveness.
levofloxacin	1	3	2	May result in decreased levofloxacin effectiveness.
levothyroxine	2	3	2	May result in hypothyroidism.
lomefloxacin	1	3	2	May result in decreased lomefloxacin effectiveness.
methyldopa	2	3	2	May result in decreased methyldopa effectiveness.
minocycline	2	3	2	May result in decreased tetracycline and iron effectiveness.
moxifloxacin	1	3	2	May result in decreased moxifloxacin effectiveness.
mycophenolate mofetil	1	3	2	May result in decreased mycophenolate mofetil efficacy.
norfloxacin	1	3	2	May result in decreased norfloxacin effectiveness.
ofloxacin	1	3	2	May result in decreased ofloxacin effectiveness.
omeprazole	1	3	2	May result in reduced non-heme iron bioavailability.
penicillamine	2	3	2	May result in decreased penicillamine effectiveness.
phytic acid containing food	1	3	2	May result in reduced iron absorption.
temafloxacin	1	3	2	May result in decreased temafloxacin effectiveness.
tetracycline	2	3	2	May result in decreased iron and tetracycline effectiveness.
trovafloxacin mesylate	1	3	2	May result in reduced efficacy of trovafloxacin.

zinc	2	3	1	May result in decreased gastrointestinal absorption of iron and/or zinc.

ISOSORBIDE MONONITRATE

sildenafil	1	1	1	May result in potentiation of hypotensive effects.
vardenafil	1	1	1	May result in potentiation of hypotensive effects.

KETOCONAZOLE

acenocoumarol	2	3	2	May result in increased risk of bleeding.
aliskiren	0	3	2	May result in increased aliskiren plasma concentrations.
almotriptan	2	3	2	May result in increased almotriptan exposure.
alosetron	0	2	1	May result in increased alosetron exposure and increased side effects.
alprazolam	0	1	1	May result in increased alprazolam concentrations and potential alprazolam toxicity (excessive sedation and prolonged hypnotic effects).
amlodipine	2	3	2	May result in increased amlodipine serum concentrations and toxicity (dizziness, hypotension, flushing, headache, peripheral edema).
amprenavir	2	3	2	May result in increased ketoconazole and/or amprenavir plasma concentrations.
anisindione	2	3	2	May result in increased risk of bleeding.

aprepitant	2	2	2	May result in increased plasma concentrations of aprepitant.
aripiprazole	2	3	2	May result in increased aripiprazole concentrations.
astemizole	2	1	2	May result in cardiotoxicity (QT prolongation, torsades de pointes, cardiac arrest).
bexarotene	0	3	2	May result in increased bexarotene exposure.
bosentan	2	3	2	May result in increased bosentan plasma concentrations.
budesonide	1	3	2	May result in increased budesonide plasma concentrations.
cerivastatin	2	2	2	May result in increased risk of myopathy or rhabdomyolysis.
chlordiazepoxide	1	3	2	May result in decreased chlordiazepoxide clearance and potentially increased chlordiazepoxide toxicity (excessive sedation and prolonged hypnotic effects).
cilostazol	2	3	2	May result in increased risk of cilostazol adverse effects (headache, diarrhea, abnormal stools).
cinacalcet	2	3	2	May result in increased bioavailability of cinacalcet and risk of hypocalcemia.
cisapride	1	1	2	May result in cardiotoxicity (QT prolongation, torsades de pointes, cardiac arrest).
conivaptan	0	1	2	May result in increased exposure to conivaptan.
conjugated estrogens	0	3	2	May result in increased plasma concentrations of estrogens.

drug	onset	severity	documentation	effect
cyclosporine	2	3	1	May result in increased risk of cyclosporine toxicity (renal dysfunction, cholestasis, paresthesias).
darifenacin	2	3	1	May result in increased darifenacin exposure and may result in increased side effects.
darunavir	0	3	1	May result in increased ketoconazole and darunavir plasma concentrations.
delavirdine	2	3	2	May result in increased serum delavirdine levels.
dicumarol	2	3	2	May result in increased risk of bleeding.
dofetilide	2	1	2	May result in increased risk of cardiotoxicity (QT prolongation, torsades de pointes, ventricular tachycardia, cardiac arrest, and/or sudden death).
dutasteride	0	3	2	May result in increased dutasteride plasma concentrations.
eplerenone	1	1	2	May result in increased eplerenone plasma concentrations and increased risk of eplerenone side effects.
Ergot Derivatives (*dihydroergotamine, ergoloid mesylates, ergonovine, ergotamine, methylergonovine, methysergide*)	0	1	2	May result in increased risk of ergotism (nausea, vomiting, vasospastic ischemia).
erlotinib	0	3	2	May result in increased erlotinib exposure.
erythromycin	2	2	2	May result in increased plasma concentrations of erythromycin and ketoconazole.

ONSET: 0 - NOT SPECIFIED 1 - RAPID 2 - DELAYED   SEVERITY: 1 - CONTRAINDICATED 2 - MAJOR 3 - MODERATE

escitalopram	0	3	2	May result in decreased ketoconazole bioavailability.
esterified estrogens	0	3	2	May result in increased plasma concentrations of estrogens.
estradiol	0	3	2	May result in increased plasma concentrations of estrogens.
eszopiclone	0	3	2	May result in increased plasma concentrations of eszopiclone.
ethanol	1	2	2	May result in disulfiram-like reaction (flushing, vomiting, increased respiratory rate, tachycardia).
felodipine	2	3	2	May result in increased felodipine serum concentrations and toxicity (dizziness, hypotension, flushing, headache, peripheral edema).
fentanyl	2	2	2	May result in increased or prolonged opioid effects (CNS depression, respiratory depression).
fosamprenavir	2	3	1	May result in increased ketoconazole plasma concentrations and increased amprenavir exposure (active metabolite of fosamprenavir).
galantamine	0	3	2	May result in increased galantamine plasma concentrations.
gefitinib	0	3	2	May result in increased gefitinib plasma concentrations.
imatinib	2	3	1	May result in increased plasma levels of imatinib.
indinavir	1	3	2	May result in increased indinavir serum concentrations and potential indinavir toxicity (nausea, headache, nephrolithiasis, asymptomatic hyperbilirubinemia).

irinotecan	0	2	2	May result in increased serum irinotecan concentrations.
isoniazid	1	3	2	May result in increased or decreased levels of ketoconazole.
isradipine	2	3	2	May result in increased isradipine serum concentrations and toxicity (dizziness, hypotension, flushing, headache, peripheral edema).
lapatinib	0	2	2	May result in increased lapatinib exposure or plasma concentrations.
levomethadyl	1	2	2	May result in increased plasma concentrations of levomethadyl and reduced active metabolites plasma concentrations.
lopinavir	2	3	1	May result in increased ketoconazole serum concentrations and increased risk of ketoconazole toxicity.
mefloquine	1	3	2	May result in increased mefloquine concentrations.
methylprednisolone	2	3	2	May result in increased risk of corticosteroid side effects (neuropsychiatric reactions, fluid and electrolyte disturbances, hypertension, hyperglycemia).
midazolam	1	2	1	May result in increased midazolam concentrations, and potentially increased midazolam toxicity (excessive sedation and prolonged hypnotic effects).
mometasone	0	3	2	May result in increased mometasone plasma concentrations.

ONSET: 0 - NOT SPECIFIED 1 - RAPID 2 - DELAYED   SEVERITY: 1 - CONTRAINDICATED 2 - MAJOR 3 - MODERATE

nevirapine	2	3	2	May result in reduced ketoconazole serum concentrations.
nicardipine	2	3	2	May result in increased nicardipine serum concentrations and toxicity (dizziness, hypotension, flushing, headache, peripheral edema).
nifedipine	2	3	2	May result in increased nifedipine serum concentrations and toxicity (dizziness, hypotension, flushing, headache, peripheral edema).
nisoldipine	2	3	2	May result in increased nisoldipine serum concentrations and toxicity (dizziness, hypotension, flushing, headache, peripheral edema).
paricalcitol	2	3	2	May result in increased plasma concentrations of paricalcitol.
phenprocoumon	2	3	2	May result in increased risk of bleeding.
pimozide	1	1	2	May result in increased risk of cardiotoxicity (QT prolongation, torsades de pointes, cardiac arrest).
pioglitazone	2	3	2	May result in increased pioglitazone serum concentrations and increased risk of hypoglycemia (CNS depression, seizures, diaphoresis, tachypnea, tachycardia, hypothermia).
prednisone	2	3	2	May result in increased risk of corticosteroid side effects (neuropsychiatric reactions, fluid and electrolyte disturbances, hypertension, hyperglycemia).
quetiapine	2	3	2	May result in increased quetiapine serum concentrations.

quinidine	2	3	2	May result in increased quinidine serum levels and toxicity (ventricular arrhythmias, hypotension, aggravated CHF).
rabeprazole	1	3	2	May result in loss of ketoconazole efficacy.
ramelteon	2	3	2	May result in increased exposure to ramelteon with increased risk of side effects.
ranolazine	0	1	2	May result in increased ranolazine steady-state plasma concentrations and increased risk of cardiotoxicity (QT prolongation, torsades de pointes, cardiac arrest).
reboxetine	1	3	2	May result in increased reboxetine bioavailability.
repaglinide	0	3	2	May result in increased repaglinide exposure and plasma concentration.
rifampin	2	3	2	May result in decreased ketoconazole and rifampin effectiveness.
rifapentine	2	3	2	May result in loss of ketoconazole efficacy.
ritonavir	2	3	2	May result in increased ketoconazole and/or ritonavir serum concentrations.
saquinavir	2	3	2	May result in significantly increased saquinavir concentrations.
sildenafil	2	3	2	May result in increased risk of prolonged sildenafil adverse effects (headache, flushing, priapism).

ONSET: 0 - NOT SPECIFIED 1 - RAPID 2 - DELAYED   SEVERITY: 1 - CONTRAINDICATED 2 - MAJOR 3 - MODERATE

simvastatin	2	2	2	May result in increased risk of myopathy or rhabdomyolysis.
sirolimus	2	2	1	May result in increased risk of sirolimus toxicity (anemia, leukopenia, thrombocytopenia, hypokalemia, diarrhea).
solifenacin	0	3	2	May result in increased plasma concentration of solifenacin.
sunitinib	2	2	2	May result in increased plasma concentrations of sunitinib and its active metabolite.
tacrolimus	2	3	2	May result in increased tacrolimus concentration.
tadalafil	1	3	2	May result in increased tadalafil bioavailability.
telithromycin	0	3	2	May result in increased telithromycin plasma concentrations.
terfenadine	1	1	1	May result in cardiotoxicity (QT prolongation, torsades de pointes, cardiac arrest).
tolbutamide	1	3	2	May result in hypoglycemia.
tolterodine	1	3	2	May result in enhanced tolterodine bioavailability in individuals with deficient cytochrome P450 2D6 activity.
trazodone	0	3	2	May result in increased trazodone plasma levels.
tretinoin	1	3	2	May result in increased risk of tretinoin toxicity.
triazolam	0	1	1	May result in increased triazolam concentrations and potential triazolam toxicity (excessive sedation and prolonged hypnotic effects).

trimetrexate	2	3	2	May result in increased trimetrexate toxicity (bone marrow suppression, renal & hepatic dysfunction, and gastrointestinal ulceration).
valdecoxib	0	3	2	May result in increased valdecoxib plasma exposure and, potentially, valdecoxib adverse effects (headache, nausea, vomiting, abdominal pain).
warfarin	2	3	2	May result in increased risk of bleeding.
zolpidem	1	3	2	May result in increased plasma concentrations and pharmacodynamic effects of zolpidem.
LAMOTRIGINE				
carbamazepine	2	3	2	May result in reduced lamotrigine efficacy, loss of seizure control, and a potential risk of neurotoxicity (nausea, vertigo, nystagmus, ataxia).
Contraceptives, Combination (*desogestrel, drospirenone, ethinyl estradiol, ethynodiol diacetate, etonogestrel, levonorgestrel, mestranol, norelgestromin, norethindrone, norgestimate, norgestrel*)	2	3	2	May result in altered (increased or decreased) plasma lamotrigine concentrations.
escitalopram	2	3	2	May result in increased risk of myoclonus.
ginkgo	2	3	2	May result in decreased anticonvulsant effectiveness.

ONSET: 0 - NOT SPECIFIED 1 - RAPID 2 - DELAYED   SEVERITY: 1 - CONTRAINDICATED 2 - MAJOR 3 - MODERATE

lopinavir	2	3	1	May result in decreased lamotrigine serum concentrations.
methsuximide	2	3	2	May result in reduced lamotrigine concentrations and possible loss of seizure control.
oxcarbazepine	2	3	2	May result in reduced lamotrigine concentrations and possible loss of seizure control.
phenobarbital	2	3	2	May result in reduced lamotrigine efficacy, loss of seizure control.
primidone	2	3	2	May result in decreased lamotrigine efficacy.
rifampin	0	3	2	May result in decreased lamotrigine exposure.
risperidone	2	3	2	May result in increased risperidone plasma concentrations and risk of adverse effects.
ritonavir	2	3	1	May result in decreased lamotrigine serum concentrations.
sertraline	2	3	2	May result in increased risk of lamotrigine toxicity (fatigue, sedation, confusion, decreased cognition).
valproic acid	2	2	1	May result in increased elimination half-life of lamotrigine leading to lamotrigine toxicity (fatigue, drowsiness, ataxia) and an increased risk of life-threatening rashes.
LANSOPRAZOLE				
acenocoumarol	2	3	2	May result in elevations in INR serum values and potentiation of anticoagulation effects.

Drug	Onset	Severity		Effect
aluminum carbonate, basic	1	3	1	May result in reduced lansoprazole bioavailability.
aluminum hydroxide	1	3	1	May result in reduced lansoprazole bioavailability.
aluminum phosphate	1	3	1	May result in reduced lansoprazole bioavailability.
Antacids (*dihydroxyaluminum aminoacetate, dihydroxyaluminum sodium carbonate, magaldrate, magnesium carbonate, magnesium hydroxide, magnesium oxide, magnesium trisilicate*)	1	3	1	May result in reduced lansoprazole bioavailability.
calcium carbonate	1	3	1	May result in reduced lansoprazole bioavailability.
cranberry	1	3	2	May result in reduced effectiveness of proton pump inhibitors.
dicumarol	2	3	2	May result in elevations in INR serum values and potentiation of anticoagulation effects.
food	1	3	2	May result in decreased lansoprazole concentrations.
phenprocoumon	2	3	2	May result in elevations in INR serum values and potentiation of anticoagulation effects.
warfarin	2	3	2	May result in elevations in INR serum values and potentiation of anticoagulation effects.

ONSET: 0 = NOT SPECIFIED 1 = RAPID 2 = DELAYED   SEVERITY: 1 = CONTRAINDICATED 2 = MAJOR 3 = MODERATE

LATANOPROST

pilocarpine	1	3	2	May result in reduced latanoprost efficacy.

LEVETIRACETAM

carbamazepine	2	3	2	May result in symptoms of carbamazepine toxicity (nystagmus, ataxia, dizziness, double vision).
ginkgo	2	3	2	May result in decreased anticonvulsant effectiveness.

LEVOFLOXACIN

Aluminum, Calcium, or Magnesium Containing Products (*aluminum carbonate, basic, aluminum hydroxide, aluminum phosphate, calcium, dihydroxyaluminum aminoacetate, dihydroxyaluminum sodium carbonate, magaldrate, magnesium carbonate, magnesium hydroxide, magnesium oxide, magnesium trisilicate*)	1	3	2	May result in decreased levofloxacin effectiveness.
Antiarrhythmic Agents, Class IA (*ajmaline, disopyramide, moricizine, pirmenol, prajmaline, procainamide, quinidine, recainam*)	1	2	2	May result in increased risk of cardiotoxicity (QT prolongation, torsades de pointes, cardiac arrest).

Drug	Onset	Severity		Description
Antiarrhythmic Agents, Class III (*amiodarone, azimilide, bretylium, dofetilide, ibutilide, sematilide, sotalol, tedisamil*)	1	2	2	May result in increased risk of cardiotoxicity (QT prolongation, torsades de pointes, cardiac arrest).
Antidiabetic Agents (*acarbose, acetohexamide, benfluorex, chlorpropamide, glicazide, glimepiride, glipizide, gliquidone, glyburide, guar gum, insulin, insulin aspart, recombinant, insulin glulisine, insulin lispro, recombinant, metformin, miglitol, repaglinide, tolazamide, tolbutamide, troglitazone*)	1	2	1	May result in changes in blood glucose and increased risk of hypoglycemia or hyperglycemia.
Corticosteroids (*betamethasone, corticotropin, cortisone, cosyntropin, deflazacort, dexamethasone, fludrocortisone, fluocortolone, hydrocortisone, methylprednisolone, paramethasone, prednisolone, prednisone, triamcinolone*)	2	3	1	May result in increased risk for tendon rupture.
droperidol	0	2	2	May result in increased risk of cardiotoxicity (QT prolongation, torsades de pointes, cardiac arrest).

fluconazole	2	2	2	May result in increased risk of QTc prolongation and torsades de pointes.
iron	1	3	2	May result in decreased levofloxacin effectiveness.
warfarin	2	3	2	May result in increased risk of bleeding.
LEVONORGESTREL				
alprazolam	2	3	2	May result in increased risk of alprazolam toxicity (CNS depression, hypotension).
amprenavir	2	3	2	May result in decreased serum concentrations of amprenavir; loss of contraceptive efficacy.
aprepitant	2	3	2	May result in reduced efficacy of combination contraceptives.
bexarotene	2	3	2	May result in decreased contraceptive effectiveness.
bosentan	2	3	2	May result in decreased contraceptive effectiveness.
carbamazepine	2	3	2	May result in decreased plasma concentrations of estrogens and in estrogen effectiveness.
fosamprenavir	2	2	1	May result in decreased serum concentrations of amprenavir, altered hormonal levels, and increased risk of hepatotoxicity.
fosphenytoin	2	3	2	May result in loss of contraceptive efficacy.
griseofulvin	2	3	1	May result in decreased contraceptive effectiveness.

lamotrigine	2	3	2	May result in altered (increased or decreased) plasma lamotrigine concentrations.
minocycline	2	3	2	May result in decreased contraceptive efficacy.
modafinil	2	3	2	May result in decreased contraceptive bioavailability and reduced contraceptive effectiveness.
mycophenolate mofetil	0	3	2	May result in decreased contraceptive exposure.
mycophenolate sodium	1	3	2	May result in decreased levonorgestrel exposure.
mycophenolic acid	1	3	2	May result in decreased levonorgestrel exposure.
nevirapine	2	3	2	May result in loss of contraceptive efficacy.
oxcarbazepine	2	3	2	May result in decreased contraceptive effectiveness.
phenobarbital	2	3	2	May result in decreased plasma concentrations of estrogens and in contraceptive effectiveness.
phenytoin	2	3	2	May result in decreased contraceptive effectiveness.
pioglitazone	2	3	2	May result in loss of contraceptive efficacy.
prednisolone	2	3	1	May result in increased risk of corticosteroid side effects (neuropsychiatric reactions, fluid and electrolyte disturbances, hypertension, hyperglycemia).
primidone	2	3	2	May result in decreased contraceptive effectiveness.
rifabutin	2	3	2	May result in increased risk of contraceptive failure.

ONSET: 0 - NOT SPECIFIED 1 - RAPID 2 - DELAYED   SEVERITY: 1 - CONTRAINDICATED 2 - MAJOR 3 - MODERATE

rifampin	2	3	1	May result in decreased plasma concentrations of estrogens and in contraceptive effectiveness.
rifapentine	2	3	2	May result in loss of oral contraceptive efficacy.
ritonavir	2	3	2	May result in altered contraceptive effectiveness and risk of side effects.
rosuvastatin	0	3	2	May result in increased exposure to ethinyl estradiol and norgestrel.
selegiline	1	3	2	May result in increased selegiline oral bioavailability and an increased risk of selegiline adverse reactions.
St. John's wort	2	3	1	May result in decreased plasma concentrations of estrogens and in contraceptive effectiveness.
tacrine	2	3	2	May result in increased risk of tacrine adverse effects.
topiramate	2	3	2	May result in reduced contraceptive efficacy.
troglitazone	2	3	2	May result in possible loss of contraception.
warfarin	2	3	2	May result in decreased or increased anticoagulant effectiveness.

LEVOTHYROXINE

Antacids (*aluminum carbonate, basic, aluminum hydroxide, aluminum phosphate, dihydroxyaluminum aminoacetate, dihydroxyaluminum sodium carbonate, fludrocortisone,*	1	3	2	May result in decreased levothyroxine effectiveness.

fluocortolone, hydrocortisone, magaldrate, magnesium carbonate, magnesium hydroxide, magnesium oxide, magnesium trisilicate)				
calcium carbonate	2	3	2	May result in decreased levothyroxine absorption.
cholestyramine	2	3	2	May result in decreased levothyroxine effectiveness.
enteral nutrition	2	3	2	May result in hypothyroidism.
Estrogens (conjugated estrogens, esterified estrogens, estradiol, estriol, estrone, estropipate)	2	3	2	May result in decreased serum-free thyroxine concentration.
imatinib	2	3	1	May result in decreased levothyroxine effectiveness and worsening of hypothyroidism.
iron	2	3	2	May result in hypothyroidism.
kelp	2	3	2	May result in increased risk of hypo- or hyperthyroidism, altered thyroid hormone dosage requirements, and inaccurate thyroid function tests used to monitor thyroid hormone therapy.
lopinavir	0	3	2	May result in loss of levothyroxine efficacy.
Oral Anticoagulants (acenocoumarol, anisindione, dicumarol, phenindione, phenprocoumon, warfarin)	2	3	2	May result in increased risk of bleeding.

ONSET: 0 – NOT SPECIFIED, 1 – RAPID, 2 – DELAYED   SEVERITY: 1 – CONTRAINDICATED, 2 – MAJOR, 3 – MODERATE

phenytoin	2	3	2	May result in decreased levothyroxine effectiveness.
rifampin	2	3	2	May result in decreased efficacy of levothyroxine.
rifapentine	2	3	2	May result in decreased levothyroxine efficacy.
ritonavir	2	3	2	May result in loss of levothyroxine efficacy.
sodium polystyrene sulfonate	1	3	2	May result in decreased absorption of levothyroxine.
soybean	2	3	2	May result in decreased effectiveness of levothyroxine.
LIDOCAINE				
amiodarone	1	2	2	May result in lidocaine toxicity (cardiac arrhythmia, seizures, coma).
amprenavir	2	2	2	May result in increased lidocaine serum concentrations and potential toxicity (hypotension, cardiac arrhythmias).
arbutamine	1	2	2	May result in increased risk of cardiac arrhythmias.
atazanavir	0	2	2	May result in increased plasma concentrations of lidocaine and an increased risk of cardiotoxicity (QT prolongation, torsades de pointes, cardiac arrest).
cimetidine	1	3	2	May result in lidocaine toxicity (neurotoxicity, cardiac arrhythmias, seizures).
creatinine measurement	0	3	2	May result in falsely increased serum creatinine values due to assay interference.
dalfopristin	2	3	2	May result in increased risk of lidocaine toxicity (neurotoxicity, cardiac arrhythmias, seizures).

fosamprenavir	2	2	2	May result in increased lidocaine serum concentrations and potential toxicity (hypotension, cardiac arrhythmias).
lopinavir	2	2	2	May result in increased lidocaine serum concentrations and potential toxicity (hypotension, cardiac arrhythmias).
metoprolol	2	2	2	May result in lidocaine toxicity (anxiety, myocardial depression, cardiac arrest).
morphine sulfate liposome	1	3	1	May result in increased peak morphine concentration.
nadolol	2	2	2	May result in lidocaine toxicity (anxiety, myocardial depression, cardiac arrest).
penbutolol	1	3	2	May result in increased volume of distribution and a prolongation of the elimination half-life of lidocaine.
phenytoin	1	2	2	May result in additive cardiac depressive effects and/or decreased lidocaine serum concentrations.
propofol	1	2	2	May result in increased hypnotic effect of propofol.
propranolol	2	2	2	May result in lidocaine toxicity (anxiety, myocardial depression, cardiac arrest).
quinupristin	2	3	2	May result in increased risk of lidocaine toxicity (neurotoxicity, cardiac arrhythmias, seizures).
St. John's wort	1	2	2	May result in increased risk of cardiovascular collapse and/or delayed emergence from anesthesia.

ONSET: 0 - NOT SPECIFIED 1 - RAPID 2 - DELAYED   SEVERITY: 1 - CONTRAINDICATED 2 - MAJOR 3 - MODERATE

succinylcholine	1	2	2	May result in succinylcholine toxicity (respiratory depression, apnea).
tocainide	1	3	2	May result in CNS toxicity (seizures).
LISINOPRIL				
ACE Inhibitors *(alacepril, benazepril, captopril, cilazapril, delapril, enalapril maleate, enalaprilat, fosinopril, imidapril, lisinopril, moexipril, pentopril, perindopril, quinapril, ramipril, spirapril, temocapril, trandolapril, zofenopril)*	2	3	2	May result in decreased antihypertensive and natriuretic effects.
aliskiren	0	3	2	May result in hyperkalemia.
aspirin	1	3	2	May result in decreased lisinopril effectiveness.
bupivacaine	2	3	2	May result in bradycardia and hypotension with loss of consciousness.
capsaicin	1	3	2	May result in increased risk of cough.
gold sodium thiomalate	0	3	2	May result in nitritoid reactions (facial flushing, nausea, vomiting, and hypotension).
lithium	2	3	2	May result in lithium toxicity (weakness, tremor, excessive thirst, confusion) and/or nephrotoxicity.
Loop Diuretics *(azosemide, bumetanide, ethacrynic acid, furosemide, piretanide, torsemide)*	1	3	2	May result in postural hypotension (first dose).

nesiritide	2	3	2	May result in increased symptomatic hypotension.
potassium	2	2	1	May result in hyperkalemia.
Potassium-Sparing Diuretics (*amiloride, canrenoate, eplerenone, spironolactone, triamterene*)	2	2	2	May result in hyperkalemia.
Thiazide Diuretics (*bemetizide, bendroflumethiazide, benthiazide, buthiazide, chlorothiazide, chlorthalidone, clopamide, cyclopenthiazide, cyclothiazide, HCTZ, hydroflumethiazide, indapamide, methyclothiazide, metolazone, polythiazide, quinethazone, trichlormethiazide, xipamide*)	1	3	2	May result in postural hypotension (first dose).
tizanidine	1	3	2	May result in potentiation of hypotensive response.
LITHIUM				
alacepril	2	3	2	May result in lithium toxicity (weakness, tremor, excessive thirst, confusion) and/or nephrotoxicity.
benazepril	2	3	2	May result in lithium toxicity (weakness, tremor, excessive thirst, confusion) and/or nephrotoxicity.
bendroflumethiazide	2	2	2	May result in increased lithium concentrations and lithium toxicity (weakness, tremor, excessive thirst, confusion).

ONSET: 0 - NOT SPECIFIED 1 - RAPID 2 - DELAYED   SEVERITY: 1 - CONTRAINDICATED 2 - MAJOR 3 - MODERATE

Drug				Interaction
benzthiazide	2	2	2	May result in increased lithium concentrations and lithium toxicity (weakness, tremor, excessive thirst, confusion).
bromfenac	2	3	2	May result in lithium toxicity (weakness, tremor, excessive thirst, confusion).
bumetanide	2	2	2	May result in increased lithium concentrations and lithium toxicity (weakness, tremor, excessive thirst, confusion).
calcitonin	1	3	2	May result in decreased lithium concentrations and loss of lithium efficacy.
carbamazepine	2	3	2	May result in additive neurotoxicity (weakness, tremor, nystagmus, asterixis).
celecoxib	2	3	2	May result in increased lithium plasma concentrations and an increased risk of lithium toxicity (weakness, tremor, excessive thirst, confusion).
chlorothiazide	2	2	2	May result in increased lithium concentrations and lithium toxicity (weakness, tremor, excessive thirst, confusion).
cilazapril	2	3	2	May result in lithium toxicity (weakness, tremor, excessive thirst, confusion) and/or nephrotoxicity.
clometacin	2	3	2	May result in lithium toxicity (weakness, tremor, excessive thirst, confusion).
cyclothiazide	2	2	2	May result in increased lithium concentrations and lithium toxicity (weakness, tremor, excessive thirst, confusion).

diclofenac	2	3	2	May result in lithium toxicity (weakness, tremor, excessive thirst, confusion).
diltiazem	2	3	2	May result in neurotoxicity, psychosis.
dipyrone	2	3	2	May result in lithium toxicity (weakness, tremor, excessive thirst, confusion).
Dopamine-2 Antagonists (*bromperidol, chlorpromazine, chlorprothixene, clozapine, domperidone, droperidol, ethopropazine, flupenthixol, fluphenazine, haloperidol, loxapine, melperone, mesoridazine, methotrimeprazine, molindone, olanzapine, penfluridol, periciazine, perphenazine, pimozide, pipamperone, pipotiazine, prochloperazine, promazine, promethazine, remoxipride, risperidone, sertindole, sulpiride, thiopropazate, thioproperazine, thioridazine, thiothixene, tiapride, trifluoperazine, triflupromazine, trimeprazine, zotepine, zuclopenthixol*)	2	2	2	May result in weakness, dyskinesias, increased extrapyramidal symptoms, encephalopathy, and brain damage.
food	1	3	2	May result in increased lithium exposure.
fosinopril	2	3	2	May result in lithium toxicity (weakness, tremor, excessive thirst, confusion) and/or nephrotoxicity.

ONSET: 0 - NOT SPECIFIED 1 - RAPID 2 - DELAYED   SEVERITY: 1 - CONTRAINDICATED 2 - MAJOR 3 - MODERATE

furosemide	2	2	2	May result in increased lithium concentrations and lithium toxicity (weakness, tremor, excessive thirst, confusion).
HCTZ	2	2	2	May result in increased lithium concentrations and lithium toxicity (weakness, tremor, excessive thirst, confusion).
hydroflumethiazide	2	2	2	May result in increased lithium concentrations and lithium toxicity (weakness, tremor, excessive thirst, confusion).
ibuprofen	2	3	2	May result in increased risk of lithium toxicity (weakness, tremor, excessive thirst, confusion).
indapamide	2	2	2	May result in increased lithium concentrations and lithium toxicity (weakness, tremor, excessive thirst, confusion).
indomethacin	2	3	2	May result in increased risk of lithium toxicity (weakness, tremor, excessive thirst, confusion).
ketoprofen	0	3	2	May result in lithium toxicity (weakness, tremor, excessive thirst, confusion).
ketorolac	2	3	2	May result in lithium toxicity (weakness, tremor, excessive thirst, confusion).
linezolid	0	2	2	May result in increased risk of serotonin syndrome (hyperthermia, hyperreflexia, myoclonus, mental status changes).
lisinopril	2	3	2	May result in lithium toxicity (weakness, tremor, excessive thirst, confusion) and/or nephrotoxicity.

losartan	2	2	2	May result in increased risk of lithium toxicity (weakness, tremor, excessive thirst, confusion).
mazindol	2	3	2	May result in lithium toxicity (weakness, tremor, excessive thirst).
mefenamic acid	2	3	2	May result in lithium toxicity (weakness, tremor, excessive thirst, confusion).
meloxicam	1	3	2	May result in elevation of plasma lithium levels and reduced renal lithium clearance.
methyclothiazide	2	2	2	May result in increased lithium concentrations and lithium toxicity (weakness, tremor, excessive thirst, confusion).
metolazone	2	2	2	May result in increased lithium concentrations and lithium toxicity (weakness, tremor, excessive thirst, confusion).
metronidazole	2	3	2	May result in elevated lithium plasma levels and lithium toxicity (weakness, tremor, excessive thirst, confusion).
perindopril	2	3	2	May result in lithium toxicity (weakness, tremor, excessive thirst, confusion) and/or nephrotoxicity.
phenelzine	2	2	2	May result in increased risk of malignant hyperpyrexia.
piroxicam	2	2	2	May result in lithium toxicity (weakness, tremor, excessive thirst, confusion).
polythiazide	2	2	2	May result in increased lithium concentrations and lithium toxicity (weakness, tremor, excessive thirst, confusion).

ONSET: 0 - NOT SPECIFIED 1 - RAPID 2 - DELAYED   SEVERITY: 1 - CONTRAINDICATED 2 - MAJOR 3 - MODERATE

quinapril	2	3	2	May result in lithium toxicity (weakness, tremor, excessive thirst, confusion) and/or nephrotoxicity.
quinethazone	2	2	2	May result in increased lithium concentrations and lithium toxicity (weakness, tremor, excessive thirst, confusion).
rofecoxib	2	3	2	May result in increased risk of lithium toxicity (weakness, tremor, excessive thirst, confusion).
sibutramine	1	2	2	May result in increased risk of serotonin syndrome (hypertension, hypothermia, myoclonus, mental status changes).
spirapril	2	3	2	May result in lithium toxicity (weakness, tremor, excessive thirst, confusion) and/or nephrotoxicity.
SSRIs (*citalopram, clovoxamine, escitalopram, femoxetine, fluoxetine, nefazodone, paroxetine, sertraline, venlafaxine, zimeldine*)	2	3	1	May result in possible increased lithium concentrations and/or an increased risk of SSRI-related serotonin syndrome (hypertension, hyperthermia, myoclonus, mental status changes).
succinylcholine	1	3	2	May result in prolongation of succinylcholine-induced neuromuscular blockade.
sulindac	2	3	2	May result in increased lithium levels.
tenidap	2	3	2	May result in increased lithium serum levels and possible lithium toxicity (weakness, tremor, excessive thirst, confusion).
tenoxicam	2	3	2	May result in lithium toxicity (weakness, tremor, excessive thirst, confusion).

tiaprofenic acid	2	3	2	May result in lithium toxicity (weakness, tremor, excessive thirst, confusion).
tolmetin	2	3	2	May result in lithium toxicity (weakness, tremor, excessive thirst, confusion).
trandolapril	2	3	2	May result in lithium toxicity (weakness, tremor, excessive thirst, confusion) and/or nephrotoxicity.
trichlormethiazide	2	2	2	May result in increased lithium concentrations and lithium toxicity (weakness, tremor, excessive thirst, confusion).
valdecoxib	2	3	2	May result in increased lithium plasma concentrations and an increased risk of lithium toxicity (weakness, tremor, excessive thirst, confusion).
valsartan	2	2	2	May result in increased risk of lithium toxicity (weakness, tremor, excessive thirst, confusion).
verapamil	2	3	2	May result in loss of mania control, neurotoxicity, bradycardia.
yohimbine	1	3	2	May result in increased risk of manic episodes.
zofenopril	2	3	2	May result in lithium toxicity (weakness, tremor, excessive thirst, confusion) and/or nephrotoxicity.

LORAZEPAM

Barbiturates (*amobarbital, aprobarbital, butabarbital, butalbital, mephobarbital, methohexital, pentobarbital, phenobarbital, primidone, secobarbital, thiopental*)	0	2	2	May result in additive respiratory depression.
Opioid Analgesics (*alfentanil, anileridine, codeine, fentanyl, hydrocodone, hydromorphone, levorphanol, meperidine, morphine, morphine sulfate liposome, oxycodone, oxymorphone, propoxyphene, remifentanil, sufentanil*)	0	2	2	May result in additive respiratory depression.
probenecid	2	3	2	May result in lorazepam toxicity.
pyrimethamine	2	3	2	May result in elevated liver function tests.
St. John's wort	2	3	2	May result in reduced BZD effectiveness.
theophylline	1	3	2	May result in decreased BZD effectiveness.
valproic acid	1	3	2	May result in increased lorazepam concentrations.

LOSARTAN

fluconazole	1	3	2	May result in decreased conversion of losartan to its active metabolite, E-3174.
indomethacin	2	3	2	May result in decreased antihypertensive effectiveness.

lithium	2	2	2	May result in increased risk of lithium toxicity (weakness, tremor, excessive thirst, confusion).
NSAIDs (aceclofenac, acemetacin, alclofenac, apazone, aspirin, benoxaprofen, bromfenac, bufexamac, carprofen, celecoxib, clometacin, clonixin, dexketoprofen, diclofenac, diflunisal, dipyrone, dofetilide, droxicam, etodolac, etofenamate, felbinac, fenbufen, fenoprofen, fentiazac, floctafenine, flufenamic acid, flurbiprofen, ibuprofen, indomethacin, indoprofen, isoxicam, ketoprofen, ketorolac, lornoxicam, meclofenamate, mefanamic acid, meloxicam, nabumetone, naproxen, niflumic acid, nimesulide, oxaprozin, oxyphenbutazone, phenylbutazone, pirazolac, piroxicam, pirprofen, propyphenazon, proquazone, rofecoxib, sulindac, suprofen, tenidap, tenoxicam, tiaprofenic acid, ticrynafen, tolmetin, zomepirac)	2	3	2	May result in decreased antihypertensive and natriuretic effects.
rifampin	2	3	2	May result in reduced losartan efficacy.

ONSET: 0 - NOT SPECIFIED 1 - RAPID 2 - DELAYED   SEVERITY: 1 - CONTRAINDICATED 2 - MAJOR 3 - MODERATE

LOVASTATIN

Drug				Description
amprenavir	2	2	2	May result in increased risk of myopathy or rhabdomyolysis.
bezafibrate	2	2	2	May result in increased risk of myopathy or rhabdomyolysis.
bosentan	1	3	2	May result in reduced plasma concentrations and reduced efficacy of lovastatin.
ciprofibrate	2	2	2	May result in increased risk of myopathy or rhabdomyolysis.
clarithromycin	2	2	2	May result in increased risk of myopathy or rhabdomyolysis.
clofibrate	2	2	2	May result in increased risk of myopathy or rhabdomyolysis.
cyclosporine	2	2	2	May result in increased risk of myopathy or rhabdomyolysis.
dalfopristin	2	2	2	May result in increased risk of myopathy or rhabdomyolysis.
diltiazem	1	3	2	May result in increased plasma concentrations of lovastatin and increased risk of myopathy or rhabdomyolysis.
erythromycin	2	2	2	May result in increased risk of myopathy or rhabdomyolysis.

	Onset	Severity		Description
fenofibrate	0	2	2	May result in increased risk of myopathy or rhabdomyolysis.
gemfibrozil	2	2	1	May result in increased risk of myopathy or rhabdomyolysis.
grapefruit juice	1	3	2	May result in increased bioavailability of lovastatin resulting in an increased risk of myopathy or rhabdomyolysis.
indinavir	2	2	2	May result in increased risk of myopathy or rhabdomyolysis.
itraconazole	2	1	2	May result in increased risk of myopathy or rhabdomyolysis.
mibefradil	2	1	2	May result in increased risk of myopathy and/or rhabdomyolysis.
nefazodone	2	2	2	May result in increased risk of myopathy or rhabdomyolysis.
nelfinavir	2	2	2	May result in increased risk of myopathy or rhabdomyolysis.
niacin	2	2	2	May result in myopathy or rhabdomyolysis.
oat bran	2	3	2	May result in reduced effectiveness of HMG CoA reductase inhibitors.
pectin	2	3	2	May result in reduced effectiveness of HMG CoA reductase inhibitors.

ONSET: 0 = NOT SPECIFIED 1 = RAPID 2 = DELAYED   SEVERITY: 1 = CONTRAINDICATED 2 = MAJOR 3 = MODERATE

quinupristin	2	2	2	May result in increased risk of myopathy or rhabdomyolysis.
ritonavir	2	2	2	May result in increased risk of myopathy or rhabdomyolysis.
saquinavir	2	2	2	May result in increased risk of myopathy or rhabdomyolysis.
St. John's wort	2	3	2	May result in reduced effectiveness of lovastatin.
telithromycin	2	2	2	May result in increased lovastatin plasma levels.
voriconazole	0	3	2	May result in increased plasma concentrations of lovastatin.

MELOXICAM

ACE Inhibitors (alacepril, benazepril, captopril, cilazapril, delapril, enalapril maleate, enalaprilat, fosinopril, imidapril, lisinopril, moexipril, pentopril, perindopril, quinapril, ramipril, spirapril, temocapril, trandolapril, zofenopril)	2	3	2	May result in decreased antihypertensive and natriuretic effects.
cholestyramine	1	3	2	May result in increased clearance of meloxicam.
clopidogrel	2	3	2	May result in increased risk of bleeding.
cyclosporine	2	3	2	May result in increased risk of cyclosporine toxicity (renal dysfunction, cholestasis, paresthesias).

danaparoid	1	2	2	May result in increased risk of bleeding and an increased risk of hematoma when neuraxial anesthesia is employed.
desvenlafaxine	0	2	2	May result in increased risk of bleeding.
lithium	1	3	2	May result in elevation of plasma lithium levels and reduced renal lithium clearance.
LMWHs (*ardeparin, certoparin, dalteparin, enoxaparin, nadroparin, parnaparin, reviparin, tinzaparin*)	1	2	2	May result in increased risk of bleeding.
Loop Diuretics (*azosemide, bumetanide, ethacrynic acid, furosemide, piretanide, torsemide*)	2	3	2	May result in decreased diuretic and antihypertensive efficacy.
Potassium-Sparing Diuretics (*amiloride, canrenoate, eplerenone, spironolactone, triamterene, torsemide*)	2	3	2	May result in reduced diuretic effectiveness, hyperkalemia, or possible nephrotoxicity.
SSRIs (*citalopram, clovoxamine, escitalopram, femoxetine, fluoxetine, nefazodone, paroxetine, sertraline, venlafaxine, zimeldine*)	0	3	2	May result in increased risk of bleeding.
Sulfonylureas (*acetohexamide, chlorpropamide, gliclazide, glimepride, glipizide, gliquidone, glyburide, tolazamide, tolbutamide*)	2	3	2	May result in increased risk of hypoglycemia.

ONSET: 0 – NOT SPECIFIED 1 – RAPID 2 – DELAYED   SEVERITY: 1 – CONTRAINDICATED 2 – MAJOR 3 – MODERATE

tacrolimus	2	2	2	May result in acute renal failure.
Thiazide Diuretics (*bemetizide, bendroflumethiazide, benzthiazide, buthiazide, chlorthalidone, clopamide, cyclopenthiazide, cyclothiazide, HCTZ, hydroflumethiazide, indapamide, methylclothiazide, metolazone, polythiazide, quinethazone, trichlormethiazide, xipamide*)	2	3	2	May result in decreased diuretic and antihypertensive efficacy.
venlafaxine	0	3	2	May result in increased risk of bleeding.
warfarin	2	3	2	May result in increased risk of bleeding.
METAXALONE				
Opioid Analgesics (*alfentanil, anileridine, codeine, fentanyl, hydrocodone, hydromorphone, levorphanol, meperidine, morphine, morphine sulfate liposome, oxycodone, oxymorphone, propoxyphene, remifentanil, sufentanil*)	0	2	2	May result in additive respiratory depression.
METFORMIN				
alatrofloxacin	1	2	1	May result in changes in blood glucose and increased risk of hypoglycemia or hyperglycemia.

Drug/Substance	Onset	Severity		Description
β-blockers (*acebutolol, alprenolol, atenolol, betaxolol, bevantolol, bisoprolol, bucindolol, carteolol, carvedilol, celiprolol, dilevalol, esmolol, labetalol, levobunolol, mepindolol, metipranolol, metoprolol, nadolol, nebivolol, oxprenolol, penbutolol, pindolol, propranolol, sotalol, talinolol, tertatolol, timolol*)	2	3	2	May result in hypoglycemia, hyperglycemia, or hypertension.
balofloxacin	1	2	1	May result in changes in blood glucose and increased risk of hypoglycemia or hyperglycemia.
bitter melon	1	3	2	May result in increased risk of hypoglycemia.
cephalexin	0	3	2	May result in increased metformin plasma levels and may increase risk of metformin side effects (nausea, vomiting, diarrhea, asthenia, headache).
cimetidine	2	2	1	May result in increased metformin plasma concentrations.
ciprofloxacin	1	2	1	May result in changes in blood glucose and increased risk of hypoglycemia or hyperglycemia.
enalapril maleate	2	3	2	May result in hyperkalemic lactic acidosis.
enalaprilat	2	3	2	May result in hyperkalemic lactic acidosis.

ONSET: 0 - NOT SPECIFIED, 1 - RAPID, 2 - DELAYED   SEVERITY: 1 - CONTRAINDICATED, 2 - MAJOR, 3 - MOD

fenugreek	1	3	2	May result in increased risk of hypoglycemia.
FLQs (alatrofloxacin, balofloxacin, ciprofloxacin, clinafloxacin, enoxacin, fleroxacin, flumequine, gatifloxacin gemifloxacin, grepafloxacin, levofloxacin, lomefloxacin, moxifloxacin, norfloxacin, ofloxacin, pefloxacin, prulifloxacin, rufloxacin, sparfloxacin, temafloxacin, tosufloxacin, trovafloxacin mesylate)	1	2	1	May result in changes in blood glucose and increased risk of hypoglycemia or hyperglycemia.
glucomannan	1	3	2	May result in increased risk of hypoglycemia.
guar gum	1	3	2	May result in decreased effectiveness of metformin.
iobitridol	1	1	2	May result in lactic acidosis and acute renal failure.
MAOIs (clorgyline, iproniazid, isocarboxazid, moclobemide, nialamide, pargyline, phenelzine, procarbazine, selegiline, toloxatone, tranylcypromine)	1	3	2	May result in excessive hypoglycemia, CNS depression, and seizures.
psyllium	1	3	2	May result in increased risk of hypoglycemia.
St. John's wort	1	3	2	May result in hypoglycemia.
topiramate	0	3	2	May result in increased metformin and topiramate exposure.

METHOCARBAMOL

Opioid Analgesics (*alfentanil, anileridine, codeine, fentanyl, hydrocodone, hydromorphone, levorphanol, meperidine, morphine, morphine sulfate liposome, oxycodone, oxymorphone, propoxyphene, remifentanil, sufentanil*)	0	2	2	May result in additive respiratory depression.

METHOTREXATE

alclofenac	2	2	2	May result in methotrexate toxicity (leukopenia, thrombocytopenia, anemia, nephrotoxicity, mucosal ulcerations).
amiodarone	2	3	2	May result in increased risk of methotrexate toxicity (leukopenia, thrombocytopenia, anemia, nephrotoxicity, mucosal ulcerations).
amoxicillin	2	2	2	May result in methotrexate toxicity.
aspirin	1	2	2	May result in methotrexate toxicity (leukopenia, thrombocytopenia, anemia, nephrotoxicity, mucosal ulcerations).
bismuth subsalicylate	2	2	2	May result in methotrexate toxicity (hemorrhage, anemia, septicemia).

ONSET: 0 = NOT SPECIFIED 1 = RAPID 2 = DELAYED   SEVERITY: 1 = CONTRAINDICATED 2 = MAJOR 3 = MODERATE

Drug				Interaction
diclofenac	2	2	2	May result in methotrexate toxicity (leukopenia, thrombocytopenia, anemia, nephrotoxicity, mucosal ulcerations).
dipyrone	2	2	2	May result in methotrexate toxicity (leukopenia, thrombocytopenia, anemia, nephrotoxicity, mucosal ulcerations).
doxycycline	1	2	2	May result in increased risk of methotrexate toxicity (leukopenia, thrombocytopenia, anemia, nephrotoxicity, mucosal ulcerations).
droxicam	2	2	2	May result in methotrexate toxicity (leukopenia, thrombocytopenia, anemia, nephrotoxicity, mucosal ulcerations).
flurbiprofen	2	2	2	May result in methotrexate toxicity (leukopenia, thrombocytopenia, anemia, nephrotoxicity, mucosal ulceration).
ibuprofen	2	2	2	May result in increased risk of methotrexate toxicity (leukopenia, thrombocytopenia, anemia, nephrotoxicity, mucosal ulcerations).
indomethacin	2	2	2	May result in increased risk of methotrexate toxicity (leukopenia, thrombocytopenia, anemia, nephrotoxicity, mucosal ulcerations).
ketoprofen	2	2	2	May result in methotrexate toxicity (leukopenia, thrombocytopenia, anemia, nephrotoxicity, mucosal ulcerations).

leflunomide	2	2	1	May result in increased risk of hepatotoxicity and bone marrow toxicity.
Live Vaccines (*bacillus of calmette and guerin vaccine, measles virus vaccine, mumps virus vaccine, poliovirus vaccine, rotavirus, rubella virus, smallpox, typhoid, varicella virus, yellow fever*)	2	2	1	May result in increased risk of infection by the live vaccine.
mercaptopurine	2	3	2	May result in mercaptopurine toxicity (nausea, vomiting, delayed leukopenia).
mezlocillin	2	2	2	May result in methotrexate toxicity.
naproxen	2	2	2	May result in increased methotrexate plasma levels and toxicity (leukopenia, thrombocytopenia, anemia, nephrotoxicity, mucosal ulcerations).
nimesulide	2	2	2	May result in methotrexate toxicity (leukopenia, thrombocytopenia, anemia, nephrotoxicity, mucosal ulcerations).
omeprazole	1	2	2	May result in increased risk of methotrexate toxicity.
Penicillins (*penicillin G, penicillin V*)	2	2	2	May result in increased risk of methotrexate toxicity.
phenytoin	1	2	2	May result in decreased phenytoin effectiveness and an increased risk of methotrexate toxicity (myelotoxicity, pancytopenia, megaloblastic anemia).

piperacillin	2	2	2	May result in methotrexate toxicity.
pirazolac	2	2	2	May result in methotrexate toxicity (leukopenia, thrombocytopenia, anemia, nephrotoxicity, mucosal ulcerations).
pristinamycin	2	2	2	May result in methotrexate toxicity (hemorrhage, anemia, septicemia).
procarbazine	2	3	2	May result in renal dysfunction.
rofecoxib	1	3	2	May result in increased risk of methotrexate toxicity (leukopenia, thrombocytopenia, anemia, nephrotoxicity, mucosal ulcerations).
sulfamethoxazole	2	2	1	May result in increased risk of methotrexate toxicity (myelotoxicity, pancytopenia, megaloblastic anemia).
sulfisoxazole	2	2	2	May result in increased risk of methotrexate toxicity (myelotoxicity, pancytopenia, megaloblastic anemia).
sulindac	2	2	2	May result in increased risk of methotrexate toxicity (leukopenia, thrombocytopenia, anemia, nephrotoxicity, mucosal ulcerations).
tamoxifen	2	2	2	May result in increased risk of thromboembolism.
tenoxicam	2	2	2	May result in methotrexate toxicity (leukopenia, thrombocytopenia, anemia, nephrotoxicity, mucosal ulcerations).

theophylline	2	3	2	May result in theophylline toxicity.
triamterene	2	2	2	May result in bone marrow suppression.
trimethoprim	2	2	1	May result in increased risk of methotrexate toxicity (myelotoxicity, pancytopenia, megaloblastic anemia).
zomepirac	2	2	2	May result in methotrexate toxicity (leukopenia, thrombocytopenia, anemia, nephrotoxicity, mucosal ulcerations).

METHYLPHENIDATE

carbamazepine	2	3	2	May result in loss of methylphenidate efficacy.

METHYLPREDNISOLONE

alcuronium	2	3	2	May result in decreased alcuronium effectiveness; prolonged muscle weakness and myopathy.
aprepitant	1	3	2	May result in increased systemic exposure to methylprednisolone.
aspirin	2	3	2	May result in increased risk of gastrointestinal ulceration and subtherapeutic aspirin serum concentrations.
atracurium	2	3	2	May result in decreased atracurium effectiveness; prolonged muscle weakness and myopathy.
carbamazepine	2	3	2	May result in decreased methylprednisolone effectiveness.
clarithromycin	2	3	2	May result in increased risk of steroid-induced adverse effects.

cyclosporine	2	3	2	May result in cyclosporine toxicity and steroid excess.
dalfopristin	2	3	2	May result in increased risk of methylprednisolone side effects (myopathy, diabetes mellitus, Cushing's syndrome).
diltiazem	1	3	2	May result in increased methylprednisolone plasma concentrations and enhanced adrenal-suppressant effects.
erythromycin	2	3	2	May result in increased risk of steroid-induced adverse effects.
FLQs (*alatrofloxacin, balofloxacin, cinoxacin, ciprofloxacin, clinafloxacin, enoxacin, fleroxacin, flumequine, gemifloxacin, grepafloxacin, levofloxacin, lomefloxacin, moxifloxacin, norfloxacin, ofloxacin, pefloxacin, prulifloxacin, rosoxacin, rufloxacin, sparfloxacin, temafloxacin, tosufloxacin, trovafloxacin*)	2	3	1	May result in increased risk for tendon rupture.
fluindione	1	2	2	May result in increased risk of bleeding.
fosphenytoin	2	3	2	May result in decreased methylprednisolone effectiveness.
gallamine	2	3	2	May result in decreased gallamine effectiveness; prolonged muscle weakness and myopathy.
hexafluorenium	2	3	2	May result in decreased hexafluorenium bromide effectiveness; prolonged muscle weakness and myopathy.

itraconazole	2	3	2	May result in increased corticosteroid plasma concentrations and an increased risk of corticosteroid side effects (myopathy, glucose intolerance, Cushing's syndrome).
ketoconazole	2	3	2	May result in increased risk of corticosteroid side effects (neuropsychiatric reactions, fluid and electrolyte disturbances, hypertension, hyperglycemia).
licorice	2	3	2	May result in increased risk of corticosteroid adverse effects.
metocurine	2	3	2	May result in decreased metocurine effectiveness; prolonged muscle weakness and myopathy.
mibefradil	1	3	2	May result in increased methylprednisolone plasma concentrations and enhanced adrenal-suppressant effects.
nefazodone	1	3	2	May result in increased methylprednisolone exposure and/or prolonged cortisol suppression.
Oral Anticoagulants (*acenocoumarol, anisindione, dicumarol, phenindione, phenprocoumon, warfarin*)	2	3	2	May result in increased risk of bleeding or diminished effects of anticoagulant.
phenobarbital	2	3	2	May result in decreased methylprednisolone effectiveness.
primidone	2	3	2	May result in decreased methylprednisolone effectiveness.
quetiapine	0	2	2	May result in decreased serum quetiapine concentrations.
quinupristin	2	3	2	May result in increased risk of methylprednisolone side effects (myopathy, diabetes mellitus, Cushing's syndrome).

ONSET 0 - NOT SPECIFIED 1 - RAPID 2 - DELAYED   CONTRAINDICATED 2 - MAJOR 3 - MODERATE

rifampin	2	3	2	May result in decreased methylprednisolone effectiveness.
rotavirus vaccine, live	2	1	1	May result in increased risk of infection by the live vaccine.
saiboku-to	2	3	2	May result in enhanced and prolonged effect of corticosteroids.
troleandomycin	2	3	2	May result in increased risk of steroid-induced adverse effects.

METOCLOPRAMIDE

cyclosporine	2	3	2	May result in increased risk of cyclosporine toxicity (renal dysfunction, cholestasis, paresthesias).
digoxin	2	3	2	May result in decreased digoxin levels.
levodopa	1	3	2	May result in increased levodopa bioavailability and an increased incidence of extrapyramidal symptoms.
linezolid	0	2	2	May result in increased risk of serotonin syndrome (hyperthermia, hyperreflexia, myoclonus, mental status changes).
mivacurium	1	3	2	May result in prolonged neuromuscular block.
sertraline	2	3	2	May result in increased risk of developing extrapyramidal symptoms.
succinylcholine	1	3	2	May result in prolonged neuromuscular blockade.
tacrolimus	2	3	2	May result in increased tacrolimus concentration.

thiopental	1	3	1	May result in enhanced hypnotic effect of thiopental.
venlafaxine	2	3	2	May result in increased risk of developing extrapyramidal symptoms.

METOPROLOL

α-1 Blockers (*alfuzosin, bunazosin, doxazosin, moxisylyte, phenosybenzamine, phentolamine, prazosin, tamsulosin, terazosin, trimazosin, urapidil*)	1	3	2	May result in exaggerated hypotensive response to the first dose of the α-blocker.
Antidiabetic Agents (*acarbose, acetohexamide, benfluorex, chlorpropamide, glicazide, glimepiride, gliquidone, glipizide, glyburide, guar gum, insulin, insulin aspart, recombinant, insulin glulisine, insulin lispro, recombinant, metformin, miglitol, repaglinide, tolazamide, tolbutamide, troglitazone*)	2	3	2	May result in hypoglycemia, hyperglycemia, or hypertension.
arbutamine	1	3	2	May result in attenuation of the response to arbutamine by the β-blocker, resulting in unreliable arbutamine test results.
bupropion	2	3	2	May result in increased plasma levels of metoprolol.

ONSET: 0 - NOT SPECIFIED, 1 - RAPID, 2 - DELAYED   SEVERITY: 1 - CONTRAINDICATED, 2 - MAJOR, 3 - MODERATE

200/METOPROLOL

INTERACTING DRUG	ONSET	SEVERITY	EVIDENCE	WARNING
CCBs, Dihydropyridine (*amlodipine, felodipine, lacidipine, lercanidipien, manidipine, nicardipine, nifedipine, nimodipine, nilvadipine, nitrendipine, nisdoldipine, prandipine*)	1	3	2	May result in hypotension and/or bradycardia.
cimetidine	1	3	2	May result in bradycardia, hypotension.
citalopram	2	3	2	May result in increased metoprolol plasma concentrations and possible loss of metoprolol cardioselectivity.
clonidine	2	2	2	May result in exaggerated clonidine withdrawal response (acute hypertension).
digoxin	2	3	2	May result in AV block and possible digoxin toxicity.
diltiazem	1	3	2	May result in increased risk of hypotension, bradycardia, AV conduction disturbances.
diphenhydramine	2	3	2	May result in increased metoprolol plasma concentration.
escitalopram	2	3	2	May result in increased metoprolol plasma concentrations and possible loss of metoprolol cardioselectivity.
fentanyl	1	2	2	May result in severe hypotension.
fluoxetine	2	3	2	May result in increased risk of metoprolol adverse effects (shortness of breath, bradycardia, hypotension, acute heart failure).
food	1	3	2	May result in increased metoprolol concentrations.

hydralazine	2	3	2	May result in metoprolol toxicity (bradycardia, fatigue, shortness of breath).
hydroxychloroquine	2	3	2	May result in increased plasma levels of metoprolol.
lidocaine	2	2	2	May result in lidocaine toxicity (anxiety, myocardial depression, cardiac arrest).
mibefradil	2	3	2	May result in hypotension, bradycardia, and AV conduction disturbances.
paroxetine	2	3	2	May result in increased risk of metoprolol adverse effects (shortness of breath, bradycardia, hypotension, acute heart failure).
phenelzine	2	3	2	May result in bradycardia.
phenobarbital	2	3	2	May result in decreased metoprolol effectiveness.
propafenone	2	3	2	May result in metoprolol toxicity (bradycardia, fatigue, shortness of breath).
propoxyphene	1	3	2	May result in increased risk of hypotension and bradycardia.
quinidine	2	3	2	May result in bradycardia, fatigue, shortness of breath.
rifampin	2	3	2	May result in decreased metoprolol effectiveness.
rifapentine	2	3	2	May result in decreased α-blocker effectiveness.

ONSET: 0 = NOT SPECIFIED 1 = RAPID 2 = DELAYED   SEVERITY: 1 = CONTRAINDICATED 2 = MAJOR 3 = MODERATE

INTERACTING DRUG	ONSET	SEVERITY	EVIDENCE	WARNING
ritonavir	2	3	2	May result in increased metoprolol serum concentrations and potential toxicity (sedation, hypotension, bradycardia, heart block).
St. John's wort	2	3	2	May result in decreased effectiveness of β-blockers.
telithromycin	0	3	2	May result in increased exposure to metoprolol.
terbinafine	2	3	2	May result in increased plasma levels of metoprolol.
thioridazine	2	3	2	May result in increased plasma levels of metoprolol.
verapamil	1	2	2	May result in hypotension, bradycardia.
METRONIDAZOLE				
amiodarone	2	2	2	May result in increased risk of cardiotoxicity (QT prolongation, torsades de pointes, cardiac arrest).
amprenavir	2	1	2	May result in increased risk of propylene glycol toxicity (seizures, tachycardia, lactic acidosis, renal toxicity, hemolysis).
busulfan	0	2	2	May result in significantly increased busulfan trough levels and an increased risk of busulfan toxicity.
carbamazepine	2	3	2	May result in increased carbamazepine serum concentrations and potential carbamazepine toxicity.
cholestyramine	1	3	2	May result in decreased metronidazole effectiveness.
cyclosporine	2	3	2	May result in increased risk of cyclosporine toxicity (nephrotoxicity, cholestasis, paresthesias).

disulfiram	1	1	2	May result in CNS toxicity (psychotic symptoms, confusion).
Ergot Derivatives (*dihydroergotamine, ergoloid mesylates, ergonovine, ergotamine, methylergonovine*)	1	1	2	May result in increased risk of ergotism (nausea, vomiting, vasospastic ischemia).
ethanol	1	2	2	May result in disulfiram-like reaction (flushing, increased respiratory rate, tachycardia) or sudden death.
fluorouracil	2	2	2	May result in increased fluorouracil serum concentrations and fluorouracil toxicity (granulocytopenia, anemia, thrombocytopenia, stomatitis, vomiting).
lithium	2	3	2	May result in elevated lithium plasma levels and lithium toxicity (weakness, tremor, excessive thirst, confusion).
milk thistle	1	3	2	May result in reduced metronidazole and active metabolite exposure.
tacrolimus	2	3	2	May result in increased serum tacrolimus concentration and increased risk of tacrolimus toxicity (nephrotoxicity, hyperglycemia, hyperkalemia).
warfarin	2	3	2	May result in increased risk of bleeding.

ONSET: 0 = NOT SPECIFIED 1 = RAPID 2 = DELAYED   SEVERITY: 1 = CONTRAINDICATED 2 = MAJOR 3 = MODERATE
EVIDENCE: 1 = EXCELLENT 2 = GOOD

MINOCYCLINE

Drug				Effect
Aluminum, Calcium, or Magnesium Containing Products (*aluminum carbonate, basic, aluminum hydroxide, aluminum phosphate, calcium, dihydroxyaluminum aminoacetate, dihydroxyaluminum sodium carbonate, magaldrate, magnesium carbonate, magnesium hydroxide, magnesium oxide, magnesium trisilicate*)	1	3	2	May result in decreased effectiveness of tetracyclines.
Contraceptives, Combination (*ethinyl estradiol, etonogestrel, mestranol, norelgestromin, norethindrone, norgestrel*)	2	3	2	May result in decreased contraceptive efficacy.
dairy food	1	3	2	May result in decreased minocycline concentrations.
iron	2	3	2	May result in decreased tetracycline and iron effectiveness.
isotretinoin	2	2	2	May result in pseudotumor cerebri (benign intracranial hypertension).
penicillin G	2	3	2	May result in decreased antibacterial effectiveness.
vitamin A	2	3	2	May result in increased risk of pseudotumor cerebri (benign intracranial hypertension).

MIRTAZAPINE

	Onset	Severity		Description
clonidine	2	2	2	May result in hypertension, decreased antihypertensive effectiveness.
diazepam	2	3	2	May result in impairment of motor skills.
ethanol	1	3	2	May result in psychomotor impairment.
linezolid	0	2	2	May result in increased risk of serotonin syndrome (hyperthermia, hyperreflexia, myoclonus, mental status changes).
MAOIs (*clorgyline, iproniazid, isocarboxazid, moclobemide, nialamide, pargyline, phenelzine, procarbazine, rasagline, selegiline, toloxatone, tranylcypromine*)	1	1	2	May result in neurotoxicity, seizures, or serotonin syndrome (hypertension, hyperthermia, myoclonus, mental status changes).
tramadol	2	2	2	May result in increased risk of serotonin syndrome (tachycardia, hyperthermia, myoclonus, mental status changes).

MOMETASONE

	Onset	Severity		Description
ketoconazole	0	3	2	May result in increased mometasone plasma concentrations.

MONTELUKAST

	Onset	Severity		Description
prednisone	2	3	2	May result in severe peripheral edema.

ONSET: 0 = NOT SPECIFIED 1 = RAPID 2 = DELAYED   SEVERITY: 1 = CONTRAINDICATED 2 = MAJOR 3 = MODERATE

INTERACTING DRUG	ONSET	SEVERITY	EVIDENCE	WARNING
MORPHINE				
Barbiturates (*amobarbital, aprobarbital, butabarbital, butalbital, mephobarbital, methohexital, pentobarbital, phenobarbital, primidone, secobarbital, thiopental*)	0	2	2	May result in additive respiratory depression.
BZDs (*adinazolam, alprazolam, bromazepam, brotizolam, chlordiazepoxide, clobazam, clonazepam, clorazepate, diazepam, estazolam, flunitrazepam, flurazepam, halazepam, ketazolam, lorazepam, lormetazepam, lormetazepam, medazepam, midazolam, nitrazepam, nordazepam, oxazepam, prazepam, temazepam, triazolam*)	0	2	2	May result in additive respiratory depression.
chloroprocaine	1	3	1	May result in antagonism of the analgesic effect of epidural morphine by epidural chloroprocaine.
cimetidine	2	2	2	May result in morphine toxicity (CNS depression, respiratory depression).
cyclosporine	2	3	2	May result in increased risk of abnormalities or malfunction of the nervous system.
esmolol	1	3	2	May result in esmolol toxicity (bradycardia, hypotension).

Drug	Onset	Severity	Doc.	Effect
Muscle Relaxants, Centrally Acting (*carisoprodol, chlorzoxazone, dantrolene, mephenesin, meprobamate, metaxalone, methocarbamol*)	0	2	2	May result in additive respiratory depression.
naltrexone	1	1	2	May result in precipitation of opioid withdrawal symptoms; decreased opioid effectiveness.
Opioid Agonists/Antagonists (*buprenorphine, butorphanol, dezocine, nalbuphine, pentazocine*)	2	2	2	May result in precipitation of withdrawal symptoms (abdominal cramps, nausea, vomiting, lacrimation, rhinorrhea, anxiety, restlessness, elevation of temperature or piloerection).
rifampin	1	3	1	May result in loss of morphine efficacy.
somatostatin	1	3	2	May result in reduced analgesic effect of morphine.
yohimbine	1	3	2	May result in increased analgesic and adverse effects of morphine.
MOXIFLOXACIN				
Antacids (*aluminum carbonate, basic, aluminum hydroxide, aluminum phosphate, dihydroxyaluminum aminoacetate, dihydroxyaluminum sodium carbonate, fludrocortisone, fluocortolone, hydrocortisone, magaldrate, magnesium carbonate, magnesium hydroxide, magnesium oxide, magnesium trisilicate*)	1	3	2	May result in decreased moxifloxacin effectiveness.

ONSET: 0 = NOT SPECIFIED, 1 = RAPID, 2 = DELAYED   SEVERITY: 1 = CONTRAINDICATED, 2 = MAJOR, 3 = MODERATE

Antidiabetic Agents (*acarbose, acetohexamide, benfluorex, chlorpropamide, glicazide, glimepiride, glipizide, gliquidone, glyburide, guar gum, insulin, insulin aspart, recombinant, insulin glulisine, insulin lispro, recombinant, metformin, miglitol, repaglinide, tolazamide, tolbutamide, troglitazone*)	1	2	1	May result in changes in blood glucose and increased risk of hypoglycemia or hyperglycemia.
Corticosteroids (*betamethasone, corticotropin, cortisone, cosyntropin, deflazacort, dexamethasone, fludrocortisone, fluocortolone, hydrocortisone, methylprednisolone, paramethasone, prednisolone, prednisone, triamcinolone*)	2	3	1	May result in increased risk for tendon rupture.
didanosine	1	3	2	May result in decreased moxifloxacin effectiveness.
droperidol	0	2	2	May result in increased risk of cardiotoxicity (QT prolongation, torsades de pointes, cardiac arrest).
erythromycin	1	2	2	May result in increased risk of cardiotoxicity (QT prolongation, torsades de pointes, cardiac arrest).
iron	1	3	2	May result in decreased moxifloxacin effectiveness.

sucralfate	1	3	2	May result in decreased moxifloxacin effectiveness.
warfarin	2	2	1	May result in increased risk of bleeding.
zinc	1	3	2	May result in decreased moxifloxacin effectiveness.
NABUMETONE				
ACE Inhibitors *(alacepril, benazepril, captopril, cilazapril, delapril, enalapril maleate, enalaprilat, fosinopril, imidapril, lisinopril, moexipril, pentopril, perindopril, quinapril, ramipril, spirapril, temocapril, trandolapril, zofenopril)*	2	3	2	May result in decreased antihypertensive and natriuretic effects.
clopidogrel	2	3	2	May result in increased risk of bleeding.
cyclosporine	2	3	2	May result in increased risk of cyclosporine toxicity (renal dysfunction, cholestasis, paresthesias).
danaparoid	1	2	2	May result in increased risk of bleeding and an increased risk of hematoma when neuraxial anesthesia is employed.
desvenlafaxine	0	2	2	May result in increased risk of bleeding.
dicumarol	2	3	2	May result in increased risk of bleeding.
ginkgo	2	2	2	May result in increased risk of bleeding.

LMWHs (*ardeparin, certoparin, dalteparin, enoxaparin, nadroparin, parnaparin, reviparin, tinzaparin*)	1	2	2	May result in increased risk of bleeding.
Loop Diuretics (*azosemide, bumetanide, ethacrynic acid, furosemide, piretanide, torsemide*)	2	3	2	May result in decreased diuretic and antihypertensive efficacy.
phenprocoumon	2	3	2	May result in increased risk of bleeding.
Potassium-Sparing Diuretics (*amiloride, canrenoate, eplerenone, spironolactone, triamterene, torsemide*)	2	3	2	May result in reduced diuretic effectiveness, hyperkalemia, or possible nephrotoxicity.
SSRIs (*citalopram, clovoxamine, femoxetine, fleinoxan, fluoxetine, nefazodone, paroxetine, sertraline, venlafaxine, zimeldine*)	0	3	2	May result in increased risk of bleeding.
Sulfonylureas (*acetohexamide, chlorpropamide, gliclazide, glimepiride, glipizide, gliquidone, glyburide, tolazamide, tolbutamide*)	2	3	2	May result in increased risk of hypoglycemia.
tacrolimus	2	2	2	May result in acute renal failure.
Thiazide Diuretics (*bemetizide, bendroflumethiazide, benzthiazide, buthiazide, chlorthiazide, chlorthalidone, clopamide, cyclopenthiazide,*	2	3	2	May result in decreased diuretic and antihypertensive efficacy.

cyclothiazide, HCTZ, hydroflumethiazide, indapamide, methyclothiazide, metolazone, polythiazide, quinethazone, trichlormethiazide, xipamide)				
venlafaxine	0	3	2	May result in increased risk of bleeding.

NALOXONE

clonidine	1	3	2	May result in hypertension.
yohimbine	1	3	1	May result in increased adverse effects.

NAPROXEN

ACE Inhibitors (alacepril, benazepril, captopril, cilazapril, delapril, enalapril maleate, enalaprilat, fosinopril, imidapril, lisinopril, moexipril, pentopril, perindopril, quinapril, ramipril, spirapril, temocapril, trandolapril, zofenopril)	2	3	2	May result in decreased antihypertensive and natriuretic effects.
clopidogrel	2	3	2	May result in increased risk of bleeding.
cyclosporine	2	3	2	May result in increased risk of cyclosporine toxicity (renal dysfunction, cholestasis, paresthesias).
danaparoid	1	2	2	May result in increased risk of bleeding and an increased risk of hematoma when neuraxial anesthesia is employed.
desvenlafaxine	0	2	2	May result in increased risk of bleeding.

ginkgo	2	2	2	May result in increased risk of bleeding.
LMWHs (*ardeparin, certoparin, dalteparin, enoxaparin, nadroparin, parnaparin, reviparin, tinzaparin*)	1	2	2	May result in increased risk of bleeding.
Loop Diuretics (*azosemide, bumetanide, ethacrynic acid, furosemide, piretanide, torsemide*)	2	3	2	May result in decreased diuretic and antihypertensive efficacy.
methotrexate	2	2	2	May result in increased methotrexate plasma levels and toxicity (leukopenia, thrombocytopenia, anemia, nephrotoxicity, mucosal ulcerations).
Potassium-Sparing Diuretics (*amiloride, canrenoate, eplerenone, spironolactone, triamterene, torsemide*)	2	3	2	May result in reduced diuretic effectiveness, hyperkalemia, or possible nephrotoxicity.
SSRIs (*citalopram, clovoxamine, femoxetine, fleinoxan, fluoxetine, nefazodone, paroxetine, sertraline, venlafaxine, zimeldine*)	2	3	2	May result in decreased diuretic and antihypertensive efficacy.
Sulfonylureas (*acetohexamide, chlorpropamide, gliclazide, glimepride, glipizide, gliquidone, glyburide, tolazamide, tolbutamide*)	2	3	2	May result in increased risk of hypoglycemia.
tacrolimus	2	2	2	May result in acute renal failure.

Thiazide Diuretics (*bemetizide, bendroflumethiazide, benzthiazide, buthiazide, chlorthiazide, chlorthalidone, clopamide, cyclopenthiazide, cyclothiazide, HCTZ, hydroflumethiazide, indapamide, methyclothiazide, metolazone, polythiazide, quinethazone, trichlormethiazide, xipamide*)	2	3	2	May result in decreased diuretic and antihypertensive efficacy.
venlafaxine	0	3	2	May result in increased risk of bleeding.
warfarin	2	2	2	May result in increased risk of bleeding.
NIACIN				
cerivastatin	2	2	2	May result in increased risk of myopathy or rhabdomyolysis.
ethanol	0	3	2	May result in increased side effects of flushing and pruritus.
lovastatin	2	2	2	May result in myopathy or rhabdomyolysis.
rosuvastatin	2	2	2	May result in increased risk of myopathy or rhabdomyolysis.
simvastatin	2	2	2	May result in increased risk of myopathy or rhabdomyolysis.

ONSET: 0 - NOT SPECIFIED, 1 - RAPID, 2 - DELAYED   SEVERITY: 1 - CONTRAINDICATED, 2 - MAJOR, 3 - MODERATE

NIFEDIPINE

Drug				Description
amiodarone	1	2	2	May result in bradycardia, atrioventricular block and/or sinus arrest.
β-Blockers (acebutolol, alprenolol, atenolol, betaxolol, bevantolol, bisoprolol, bucindolol, carteolol, carvedilol, celiprolol, dilevalol, esmolol, labetalol, levobunolol, mepindolol, metipranolol, metoprolol, nadolol, nebivolol, oxprenolol, penbutolol, pindolol, propranolol, sotalol, talinolol, tertatolol, timolol)	1	3	2	May result in hypotension and/or bradycardia.
cimetidine	2	3	2	May result in increased nifedipine serum concentrations and toxicity (headache, peripheral edema, hypotension, tachycardia).
dalfopristin	2	3	2	May result in increased risk of nifedipine toxicity (headache, peripheral edema, hypotension, tachycardia).
diltiazem	1	3	2	May result in nifedipine toxicity (headache, peripheral edema, hypotension, tachycardia).
doxazosin	2	3	2	May result in increased plasma concentration of nifedipine, which may result in increased risk of hypotension.
fentanyl	1	2	2	May result in severe hypotension.

	ONSET		SEVERITY	

fluconazole	2	3	2	May result in increased nifedipine serum concentrations and toxicity (dizziness, hypotension, flushing, headache, peripheral edema).
ginkgo	2	3	2	May result in increased risk of nifedipine side effects.
ginseng	2	3	2	May result in increased risk of nifedipine side effects.
grapefruit juice	1	3	1	May result in severe hypotension, myocardial ischemia, increased vasodilator side effects.
indinavir	0	3	2	May result in increased plasma concentrations of CCB.
itraconazole	2	3	2	May result in increased nifedipine serum concentrations and toxicity (dizziness, hypotension, flushing, headache, peripheral edema).
ketoconazole	2	3	2	May result in increased nifedipine serum concentrations and toxicity (dizziness, hypotension, flushing, headache, peripheral edema).
magnesium	1	3	2	May result in hypotension.
mibefradil	1	2	2	May result in severe bradycardia and hypotension.
micafungin	0	3	2	May result in increased nifedipine exposure.
nafcillin	1	3	2	May result in decreased nifedipine efficacy.
nevirapine	0	3	2	May result in decreased plasma concentrations of nifedipine.

ONSET: 0 - NOT SPECIFIED, 1 - RAPID, 2 - DELAYED   SEVERITY: 1 - CONTRAINDICATED, 2 - MAJOR, 3 - MODER...

phenytoin	2	3	2	May result in increased risk of phenytoin toxicity (ataxia, hyperreflexia, nystagmus, tremor).
quinidine	2	3	2	May result in decreased quinidine effectiveness and/or an increased risk of nifedipine adverse effects (headache, peripheral edema, hypotension, tachycardia).
quinupristin	2	3	2	May result in increased risk of nifedipine toxicity (headache, peripheral edema, hypotension, tachycardia).
rifampin	2	3	2	May result in decreased nifedipine effectiveness.
rifapentine	2	3	2	May result in decreased CCB effectiveness.
saquinavir	1	3	2	May result in increased risk of nifedipine toxicity (headache, peripheral edema, hypotension, tachycardia).
St. John's wort	2	3	2	May result in reduced bioavailability of CCB.
tacrolimus	2	3	1	May result in increased tacrolimus concentration.
vincristine	2	3	2	May result in increased risk of vincristine toxicity (neuropathy, delirium, seizures).
vincristine liposome	2	3	2	May result in increased risk of vincristine toxicity (neuropathy, delirium, seizures).
voriconazole	0	3	2	May result in increased plasma concentrations of CCB.
NITROFURANTOIN				
fluconazole	2	2	2	May result in increased risk of hepatic and pulmonary toxicity.

NITROGLYCERIN

acetylcysteine	1	3	1	May result in enhanced hypotension and nitroglycerin-induced headache.
alteplase, recombinant	1	2	2	May result in less coronary artery reperfusion, longer time to reperfusion, and more coronary artery reocclusion.
aspirin	1	3	2	May result in increased nitroglycerin concentrations and additive platelet function depression.
dihydroergotamine	1	3	2	May result in dihydroergotamine toxicity (peripheral ischemia, paresthesias, nausea, vomiting).
pancuronium	2	3	2	May result in increased pancuronium duration of action.
sildenafil	1	1	1	May result in potentiation of hypotensive effects.
vardenafil	1	1	1	May result in potentiation of hypotensive effects.

NORELGESTROMIN

alprazolam	2	3	2	May result in increased risk of alprazolam toxicity (CNS depression, hypotension).
amoxicillin	2	3	2	May result in decreased contraceptive effectiveness.
ampicillin	2	3	2	May result in decreased contraceptive effectiveness.
amprenavir	2	3	2	May result in decreased serum concentrations of amprenavir; loss of contraceptive efficacy.

ONSET: 0 - NOT SPECIFIED 1 - RAPID 2 - DELAYED   SEVERITY: 1 - CONTRAINDICATED 2 - MAJOR 3 - MODERATE

bacampicillin	2	3	2	May result in decreased contraceptive effectiveness.
betamethasone	2	3	2	May result in increased corticosteroid effects.
bexarotene	2	3	2	May result in decreased contraceptive effectiveness.
bosentan	2	3	2	May result in decreased contraceptive effectiveness.
caffeine	1	3	2	May result in enhanced CNS stimulation.
carbamazepine	2	3	2	May result in decreased plasma concentrations of estrogens and in estrogen effectiveness.
cyclosporine	2	3	2	May result in increased risk of cyclosporine toxicity (renal dysfunction, cholestasis, paresthesias).
doxycycline	2	3	2	May result in decreased contraceptive effectiveness.
fosamprenavir	2	2	1	May result in decreased serum concentrations of amprenavir, altered hormonal levels, and an increased risk of hepatotoxicity.
fosphenytoin	2	3	2	May result in decreased contraceptive effectiveness.
griseofulvin	2	3	1	May result in decreased contraceptive effectiveness.
lamotrigine	2	3	2	May result in altered (increased or decreased) plasma lamotrigine concentrations.
licorice	2	3	2	May result in increased risk of fluid retention and elevated blood pressure.

modafinil	2	3	2	May result in decreased contraceptive bioavailability and reduced contraceptive effectiveness.
mycophenolate sodium	1	3	2	May result in decreased levonorgestrel exposure.
mycophenolic acid	1	3	2	May result in decreased levonorgestrel exposure.
oxcarbazepine	2	3	2	May result in decreased contraceptive effectiveness.
oxytetracycline	2	3	2	May result in decreased contraceptive effectiveness.
phenobarbital	2	3	2	May result in decreased plasma concentrations of estrogens and in contraceptive effectiveness.
phenytoin	2	3	2	May result in decreased contraceptive effectiveness.
prednisolone	2	3	1	May result in increased risk of corticosteroid side effects (neuropsychiatric reactions, fluid and electrolyte disturbances, hypertension, hyperglycemia).
primidone	2	3	2	May result in decreased contraceptive effectiveness.
rifabutin	2	3	2	May result in increased risk of contraceptive failure.
rifampin	2	3	1	May result in decreased plasma concentrations of estrogens and in contraceptive effectiveness.
ritonavir	2	3	2	May result in altered contraceptive effectiveness and risk of side effects.
rosuvastatin	0	3	2	May result in increased exposure to ethinyl estradiol and norgestrel.

ONSET: 0 – NOT SPECIFIED 1 – RAPID 2 – DELAYED   SEVERITY: 1 – CONTRAINDICATED 2 – MAJOR 3 – MODERATE

St. John's wort	2	3	1	May result in decreased plasma concentrations of estrogens and in contraceptive effectiveness.
tetracycline	2	3	2	May result in decreased contraceptive effectiveness.
topiramate	2	3	2	May result in reduced contraceptive efficacy.
troleandomycin	2	3	1	May result in altered contraceptive effectiveness and risk of hepatotoxicity.
warfarin	2	3	2	May result in decreased or increased anticoagulant effectiveness.
NORGESTIMATE				
alprazolam	2	3	2	May result in increased risk of alprazolam toxicity (CNS depression, hypotension).
amprenavir	2	3	2	May result in decreased serum concentrations of amprenavir; loss of contraceptive efficacy.
bexarotene	2	3	2	May result in decreased contraceptive effectiveness.
bosentan	2	3	2	May result in decreased contraceptive effectiveness.
fosamprenavir	2	2	1	May result in decreased serum concentrations of amprenavir, altered hormonal levels, and an increased risk of hepatotoxicity.
lamotrigine	2	3	2	May result in altered (increased or decreased) plasma lamotrigine concentrations.

modafinil	2	3	2	May result in decreased contraceptive bioavailability and reduced contraceptive effectiveness.
prednisolone	2	3	1	May result in increased risk of corticosteroid side effects (neuropsychiatric reactions, fluid and electrolyte disturbances, hypertension, hyperglycemia).
rosuvastatin	0	3	2	May result in increased exposure to ethinyl estradiol and norgestrel.
St. John's wort	2	3	1	May result in decreased plasma concentrations of estrogens and in contraceptive effectiveness.
topiramate	2	3	2	May result in reduced contraceptive efficacy.
NORETHINDRONE				
alprazolam	2	3	2	May result in an increased risk of alprazolam toxicity (CNS depression, hypotension).
amoxicillin	2	3	2	May result in decreased contraceptive effectiveness.
ampicillin	2	3	2	May result in decreased contraceptive effectiveness.
amprenavir	2	3	2	May result in decreased serum concentrations of amprenavir; loss of contraceptive efficacy.
aprepitant	0	3	2	May result in reduced efficacy of combination contraceptives.
bacampicillin	2	3	2	May result in decreased contraceptive effectiveness.

ONSET: 0 – NOT SPECIFIED 1 – RAPID 2 – DELAYED   SEVERITY: 1 – CONTRAINDICATED 2 – MAJOR 3 – MODERATE

betamethasone	2	3	2	May result in increased corticosteroid effects.
bexarotene	2	3	2	May result in decreased contraceptive effectiveness.
bosentan	2	3	2	May result in decreased contraceptive effectiveness.
caffeine	1	3	2	May result in enhanced CNS stimulation.
carbamazepine	2	3	2	May result in decreased plasma concentrations of estrogens and decreased estrogen effectiveness.
colesevelam	1	3	2	May result in decreased contraceptive effectiveness.
cyclosporine	2	3	2	May result in increased risk of cyclosporine toxicity (renal dysfunction, cholestasis, paresthesias).
doxycycline	2	3	2	May result in decreased contraceptive effectiveness.
fosamprenavir	0	3	1	May result in altered hormonal levels and an increased risk of liver enzyme elevations.
fosaprepitant	2	3	2	May result in reduced efficacy of combination contraceptives.
fosphenytoin	2	3	2	May result in decreased contraceptive effectiveness.
griseofulvin	2	3	1	May result in decreased contraceptive effectiveness.
lamotrigine	2	3	1	May result in altered (increased or decreased) plasma lamotrigine concentrations.
licorice	2	3	2	May result in increased risk of fluid retention and elevated blood pressure.
minocycline	2	3	2	May result in decreased contraceptive efficacy.

modafinil	2	3	2	May result in decreased contraceptive bioavailability and reduced contraceptive effectiveness.
mycophenolate mofetil	0	3	2	May result in decreased contraceptive exposure.
mycophenolic acid	1	3	2	May result in decreased levonorgestrel exposure.
nelfinavir	2	3	2	May result in contraceptive failure.
nevirapine	2	3	2	May result in loss of contraceptive efficacy.
oxcarbazepine	2	3	2	May result in decreased contraceptive effectiveness.
oxytetracycline	2	3	2	May result in decreased contraceptive effectiveness.
phenobarbital	2	3	2	May result in decreased plasma concentrations of estrogens and decreased contraceptive effectiveness.
phenytoin	2	3	2	May result in decreased contraceptive effectiveness.
pioglitazone	2	3	2	May result in loss of contraceptive efficacy.
prednisolone	2	3	1	May result in increased risk of corticosteroid side effects (neuropsychiatric reactions, fluid and electrolyte disturbances, hypertension, hyperglycemia).
primidone	2	3	2	May result in decreased contraceptive effectiveness.
rifabutin	2	3	2	May result in increased risk of contraceptive failure.

rifampin	2	3	1	May result in decreased plasma concentrations of estrogens and decreased contraceptive effectiveness.
rifapentine	2	3	2	May result in loss of oral contraceptive efficacy.
ritonavir	2	3	2	May result in altered contraceptive effectiveness and risk of side effects.
rosuvastatin	0	3	2	May result in increased exposure to ethinyl estradiol and norgestrel.
selegiline	1	3	2	May result in an increase in selegiline oral bioavailability and an increased risk of selegiline adverse reactions.
St. John's wort	2	3	1	May result in decreased plasma concentrations of estrogens and decreased contraceptive effectiveness.
tetracycline	2	3	2	May result in decreased contraceptive effectiveness.
topiramate	2	3	2	May result in reduced contraceptive efficacy.
troglitazone	2	3	2	May result in possible loss of contraception.
troleandomycin	2	3	1	May result in altered contraceptive effectiveness and risk of hepatotoxicity.
valdecoxib	0	3	2	May result in increased exposure of norethindrone and ethinyl estradiol.

voriconazole	2	3	1	May result in increased levels of voriconazole and of ethinyl estradiol and norethindrone.
warfarin	2	3	2	May result in decreased or increased anticoagulant effectiveness.

NORTRIPTYLINE

acenocoumarol	2	3	2	May result in increased risk of bleeding.
amprenavir	2	2	2	May result in increased tricyclic serum concentrations and potential toxicity (anticholinergic effects, sedation, confusion, cardiac arrhythmias).
Antiarrhythmic Agents, Class IA (ajmaline, disopyramide, hydroquinidine, pirmenol, prajmaline, procainamide, quinidine)	0	2	2	May result in increased risk of cardiotoxicity (QT prolongation, torsades de pointes, cardiac arrest).
arbutamine	1	3	2	May result in unreliable arbutamine test results.
atomoxetine	0	3	2	May result in increased atomoxetine steady-state plasma concentrations.
bupropion	2	3	2	May result in increased plasma levels of nortriptyline.
carbamazepine	2	3	2	May result in decreased nortriptyline effectiveness.
cimetidine	2	3	2	May result in nortriptyline toxicity (dry mouth, blurred vision, urinary retention).

clonidine	2	2	2	May result in decreased antihypertensive effectiveness.
dicumarol	2	3	2	May result in increased risk of bleeding.
duloxetine	0	3	2	May result in increased tricyclic antidepressant serum concentrations and potential toxicity (anticholinergic effects, sedation, confusion, cardiac arrhythmias).
enflurane	0	2	2	May result in increased risk of cardiotoxicity (QT prolongation, torsades de pointes, cardiac arrest) and increased risk of seizure activity.
fluconazole	0	2	2	May result in increased risk of nortriptyline toxicity and increased risk of cardiotoxicity (QT prolongation, torsades de pointes, cardiac arrest).
fluoxetine	0	2	2	May result in tricyclic antidepressant toxicity (dry mouth, urinary retention, sedation) and increased risk of cardiotoxicity (QT prolongation, torsades de pointes, cardiac arrest).
fosamprenavir	2	2	2	May result in increased tricyclic agent serum concentrations and potential toxicity (anticholinergic effects, sedation, confusion, cardiac arrhythmias).
grepafloxacin	2	1	2	May result in increased risk of cardiotoxicity (QT prolongation, torsades de pointes, cardiac arrest).

halofantrine	2	2	2	May result in increased risk of cardiotoxicity (QT prolongation, torsades de pointes, cardiac arrest).
iproniazid	2	2	2	May result in neurotoxicity, seizures, or serotonin syndrome (hypertension, hyperthermia, myoclonus, mental status changes).
moclobemide	2	1	2	May result in neurotoxicity, seizures, or serotonin syndrome (hypertension, hyperthermia, myoclonus, mental status changes).
nefopam	1	2	2	May result in increased risk of seizures.
nialamide	2	2	2	May result in neurotoxicity, seizures, or serotonin syndrome (hypertension, hyperthermia, myoclonus, mental status changes).
pargyline	2	2	2	May result in neurotoxicity, seizures, or serotonin syndrome (hypertension, hyperthermia, myoclonus, mental status changes).
paroxetine	2	3	2	May result in nortriptyline toxicity (dry mouth, sedation, urinary retention).
phenprocoumon	2	3	2	May result in increased risk of bleeding.
prochlorperazine	1	2	2	May result in increased risk of cardiotoxicity (QT prolongation, torsades de pointes, cardiac arrest).

rifapentine	2	3	2	May result in decreased nortriptyline efficacy.
s-adenosylmethionine	2	3	2	May result in increased risk of serotonin syndrome (hypertension, hyperthermia, myoclonus, mental status changes).
sertraline	2	2	2	May result in elevated nortriptyline serum levels or possible serotonin syndrome (hypertension, hyperthermia, myoclonus, mental status changes).
sulfamethoxazole	0	2	2	May result in increased risk of cardiotoxicity (QT prolongation, torsades de pointes, cardiac arrest).
Sympathomimetics, Direct Acting (epinephrine, etilefrine, methoxamine, midrodrine norepinephrine, oxilofrine, phenylephrine)	1	2	2	May result in hypertension, cardiac arrhythmias, and tachycardia.
terbinafine	2	3	2	May result in increased risk of nortriptyline toxicity (fatigue, vertigo, loss of appetite).
toloxatone	2	2	2	May result in neurotoxicity, seizures, or serotonin syndrome (hypertension, hyperthermia, myoclonus, mental status changes).
trifluoperazine	1	2	2	May result in increased risk of cardiotoxicity (QT prolongation, torsades de pointes, cardiac arrest).

trimethoprim	0	2	2	May result in increased risk of cardiotoxicity (QT prolongation, torsades de pointes, cardiac arrest).
valproic acid	2	3	2	May result in increased serum nortriptyline levels.
OLANZAPINE				
betel nut	2	3	2	May result in increased extrapyramidal side effects of olanzapine (difficulty with movement or abnormal movement of muscles).
carbamazepine	1	3	2	May result in reduced olanzapine efficacy.
ciprofloxacin	2	3	2	May result in increased risk of olanzapine toxicity (increased sedation, orthostatic hypotension).
clomipramine	2	2	2	May result in increased risk of seizures.
fluvoxamine	2	3	2	May result in increased risk of olanzapine adverse effects.
haloperidol	2	3	2	May result in increased risk of parkinsonism (cogwheeling rigidity, unstable gait).
lithium	2	2	2	May result in weakness, dyskinesias, increased extrapyramidal symptoms, encephalopathy, and brain damage.

OLMESARTAN

NSAIDs (aceclofenac, acemetacin, alclofenac, apazone, aspirin, benoxaprofen, bromfenac, bufexamac, carprofen, celecoxib, clometacin, clonixin, dexketoprofen, diclofenac, diflunisal, dipyrone, dofetilide, droxicam, etodolac, etofenamate, felbinac, fenbufen, fenoprofen, fentiazac, floctafenine, flufenamic acid, flurbiprofen, ibuprofen, indomethacin, indoprofen, isoxicam, ketoprofen, ketorolac, lornoxicam, meclofenamate, mefenamic acid, meloxicam, nabumetone, naproxen, niflumic acid, nimesulide, oxaprozin, oxyphenbutazone, phenylbutazone, pirazolac, piroxicam, pirprofen, propyphenazon, proquazone, rofecoxib, sulindac, suprofen, tenidap, tenoxicam, tiaprofenic acid, ticrynafen, tolmetin, zomepirac)	2	3	2	May result in decreased antihypertensive and natriuretic effects.

OMEPRAZOLE

atazanavir	0	2	1	May result in decreased atazanavir plasma concentrations and risk of diminished therapeutic effect of atazanavir.

	Onset	Severity	Documentation	
carbamazepine	2	3	2	May result in increased risk of carbamazepine toxicity.
cilostazol	2	3	2	May result in increased risk of cilostazol adverse effects (headache, diarrhea, abnormal stools).
clorazepate	2	2	2	May result in increased risk of clorazepate toxicity.
cranberry	1	3	2	May result in reduced effectiveness of proton pump inhibitors.
digoxin	1	3	2	May result in increased risk of digoxin toxicity (nausea, vomiting, arrhythmias).
disulfiram	2	3	2	May result in disulfiram toxicity (confusion, disorientation, psychotic changes).
ginkgo	1	3	2	May result in reduced omeprazole effectiveness.
iron	1	3	2	May result in reduced non-heme iron bioavailability.
methotrexate	1	2	2	May result in increased risk of methotrexate toxicity.
St. John's wort	1	3	2	May result in decreased serum concentration of omeprazole.
triazolam	2	3	2	May result in BZD toxicity (CNS depression, ataxia, lethargy).
voriconazole	0	3	2	May result in increased plasma concentrations of omeprazole.
warfarin	2	3	2	May result in elevations of INR serum values and potentiation of anticoagulant effects.

ONSET: 0 - NOT SPECIFIED 1 - RAPID 2 - DELAYED   SEVERITY: 1 - CONTRAINDICATED 2 - MAJOR 3 - MODERATE

OSELTAMIVIR

none reported

OXYCODONE

Barbiturates (amobarbital, aprobarbital, butabarbital, butalbital, mephobarbital, methohexital, pentobarbital, phenobarbital, secobarbital, thiopental)	0	2	2	May result in additive respiratory depression.
BZDs (adinazolam, alprazolam, bromazepam, brotizolam, chlordiazepoxide, clobazam, clonazepam, clorazepate, diazepam, estazolam, flunitrazepam, flurazepam, halazepam, ketazolam, lorazepam, lormetazepam, lormetazepam, medazepam, midazolam, nitrazepam, nordazepam, oxazepam, prazepam, temazepam, triazolam)	0	2	2	May result in additive respiratory depression.
escitalopram	2	2	2	May result in increased risk of serotonin syndrome (tachycardia, hyperthermia, myoclonus, mental status changes).
fluvoxamine	2	2	2	May result in increased risk of serotonin syndrome (tachycardia, hyperthermia, myoclonus, mental status changes).

Drug			Interaction
MAOIs (*clorgyline, iproniazid, isocarboxazid, moclobemide, nialamide, pargyline, phenelzine, procarbazine, selegiline, toloxatone, tranylcypromine*)	2	2	2	May result in CNS depression (sedation, lethargy, speech difficulties).
Muscle Relaxants, Centrally Acting (*carisoprodol, chlorzoxazone, dantrolene, mephenesin, meprobamate, metazalone, methocarbomol*)	0	2	2	May result in additive respiratory depression.
naltrexone	1	1	2	May result in precipitation of opioid withdrawal symptoms; decreased opioid effectiveness.
Opioid Agonists/Antagonists (*buprenorphine, butorphanol, dezocine, nalbuphine, pentazocine*)	0	2	2	May result in additive respiratory depression.
Opioid Analgesics (*alfentanil, anileridine, codeine, fentanyl, hydrocodone, hydromorphone, levorphanol, meperidine, morphine, morphine sulfate liposome, oxycodone, oxymorphone, propoxyphene, remifentanil, sufentanil*)	0	2	2	May result in additive respiratory depression.
sertraline	2	2	2	May result in increased risk of serotonin syndrome (tachycardia, hyperthermia, myoclonus, mental status changes).

ONSET: 0 = NOT SPECIFIED, 1 = RAPID, 2 = DELAYED   SEVERITY: 1 = CONTRAINDICATED, 2 = MAJOR, 3 = MODERATE

PANTOPRAZOLE

cranberry	1	3	2	May result in reduced effectiveness of proton pump inhibitors.
itraconazole	2	3	2	May result in loss of itraconazole efficacy.
warfarin	0	3	2	May result in increased INR and prothrombin time.

PAROXETINE

amitriptyline	2	3	2	May result in amitriptyline toxicity (dry mouth, sedation, urinary retention).
amoxapine	2	3	2	May result in amoxapine toxicity (dry mouth, sedation, urinary retention).
Anticoagulants (*abciximab, acenocoumarol, ancrod, anisindione, antithrombin III human, bivalirudin, cilostazol, clopidogrel, danaparoid, defibrotide, dermatan sulfate, dicumarol, eptifibatide, fondaparinux, lamifiban, pentosan polysulfate sodium, phenindione, phenprocoumon, sibrafiban, warfarin, xemilofiban*)	0	2	2	May result in increased risk of bleeding.
Antiplatelet Agents (*abciximab, anagrelide, aspirin, cilostazol, clopidogrel, dipyridamole, epoprostenol, eptifibatide, iloprost,*	0	2	2	May result in increased risk of bleeding.

lamifiban, lexipafant, sulfinpyrazone, sulodexide, ticlopidine, tirofiban, xemilofiban)				
aprepitant	2	3	2	May result in decreased AUC and Cmax of aprepitant and paroxetine.
bupropion	2	3	2	May result in increased plasma levels of paroxetine.
cimetidine	2	3	2	May result in increased paroxetine serum concentrations and possibly paroxetine toxicity (dizziness, somnolence, nausea, headache).
clarithromycin	2	3	2	May result in increased risk of serotonin syndrome (hypertension, hyperthermia, myoclonus, mental status changes).
clomipramine	0	3	2	May result in clomipramine toxicity (dry mouth, sedation, urinary retention).
clorgyline	1	1	2	May result in CNS toxicity or serotonin syndrome (hypertension, hyperthermia, myoclonus, mental status changes).
clozapine	2	3	2	May result in increased risk of clozapine toxicity (sedation, seizures, hypotension).
cyproheptadine	2	3	2	May result in reduced paroxetine efficacy.

ONSET: 0 - NOT SPECIFIED 1 - RAPID 2 - DELAYED   SEVERITY: 1 - CONTRAINDICATED 2 - MAJOR 3 - MODERATE

darunavir	0	3	1	May result in decreased paroxetine exposure and plasma concentrations.
desipramine	2	3	2	May result in increased plasma concentrations of desipramine and in related side effects (dry mouth, sedation).
dextromethorphan	1	2	2	May result in possible dextromethorphan toxicity (nausea, vomiting, blurred vision, hallucinations) or serotonin syndrome (hypertension, hyperthermia, myoclonus, mental status changes).
dothiepin	2	3	2	May result in dothiepin toxicity (dry mouth, sedation, urinary retention).
doxepin	2	3	2	May result in doxepin toxicity (dry mouth, sedation, urinary retention).
duloxetine	0	3	2	May result in increased duloxetine and paroxetine serum concentrations and risk of adverse effects.
eletriptan	2	2	2	May result in increased risk of serotonin syndrome.
encainide	1	3	2	May result in increased risk of encainide toxicity (cardiac arrhythmia).
flecainide	2	3	2	May result in increased risk of flecainide toxicity (cardiac arrhythmia).
fluoxetine	2	3	2	May result in fluoxetine toxicity (dry mouth, sedation, urinary retention).

Drug	Onset	Severity	Documentation	Description
fluphenazine	2	3	2	May result in increased risk of developing acute parkinsonism.
fosamprenavir	0	3	2	May result in decreased paroxetine plasma levels.
fosphenytoin	2	3	2	May result in reduced paroxetine efficacy.
frovatriptan	2	2	2	May result in increased risk of serotonin syndrome.
galantamine	0	3	2	May result in increased galantamine plasma concentrations.
ginkgo	2	3	2	May result in increased risk of serotonin syndrome (hypertension, hyperthermia, myoclonus, mental status changes).
imipramine	2	3	2	May result in imipramine toxicity (dry mouth, sedation, urinary retention).
iproniazid	1	1	2	May result in CNS toxicity or serotonin syndrome (hypertension, hyperthermia, myoclonus, mental status changes).
linezolid	1	2	2	May result in CNS toxicity or serotonin syndrome (hypertension, hyperthermia, myoclonus, mental status changes).
lithium	2	3	1	May result in possible increased lithium concentrations and/or an increased risk of SSRI-related serotonin syndrome (hypertension, hyperthermia, myoclonus, mental status changes).

ONSET: 0 - NOT SPECIFIED 1 - RAPID 2 - DELAYED   SEVERITY: 1 - CONTRAINDICATED 2 - MAJOR 3 - MODERATE

lofepramine	2	3	2	May result in lofepramine toxicity (dry mouth, sedation, urinary retention).
metoprolol	2	3	2	May result in increased risk of metoprolol adverse effects (shortness of breath, bradycardia, hypotension, acute heart failure).
moclobemide	1	1	2	May result in CNS toxicity or serotonin syndrome (hypertension, hyperthermia, myoclonus, mental status changes).
naratriptan	2	2	2	May result in increased risk of serotonin syndrome.
nefazodone	1	2	2	May result in CNS toxicity or serotonin syndrome (hypertension, hyperthermia, myoclonus, mental status changes).
nialamide	1	1	2	May result in CNS toxicity or serotonin syndrome (hypertension, hyperthermia, myoclonus, mental status changes).
nortriptyline	2	3	2	May result in nortriptyline toxicity (dry mouth, sedation, urinary retention).
NSAIDs (aceclofenac, acemetacin, alclofenac, apazone, benoxaprofen, bromfenac, bufexamac, carprofen, celecoxib, clometacin, clonixin, dexketoprofen, diclofenac, diflunisal, dipyrone, dofetilide, droxicam, etodolac,	0	3	2	May result in increased risk of bleeding.

etofenamate, felbinac, fenbufen, fenoprofen, fentiazac, floctafenine, flufenamic acid, flurbiprofen, ibuprofen, indomethacin, indoprofen, isoxicam, ketoprofen, ketorolac, lornoxicam, meclofenamate, mefanamic acid, meloxicam, nabumetone, naproxen, niflumic acid, nimesulide, oxaprozin, oxyphenbutazone, phenylbutazone, pirazolac, piroxicam, pirprofen, propyphenazon, proquazone, rofecoxib, sulindac, suprofen, tenidap, tenoxicam, tiaprofenic acid, ticrynafen, tolmetin, zomepirac)				
pargyline	1	1	2	May result in CNS toxicity or serotonin syndrome (hypertension, hyperthermia, myoclonus, mental status changes).
perhexiline	2	3	2	May result in increased risk of perhexiline toxicity (ataxia, lethargy, nausea).
perphenazine	1	3	2	May result in increased plasma concentrations and side effects of perphenazine.
phenytoin	2	3	2	May result in reduced phenytoin efficacy; reduced paroxetine efficacy.

ONSET: 0 – NOT SPECIFIED, 1 – RAPID, 2 – DELAYED   SEVERITY: 1 – CONTRAINDICATED, 2 – MAJOR, 3 – MODERATE

Drug				Description
pimozide	1	1	2	May result in increased risk of pimozide toxicity including cardiotoxicity (QT prolongation, torsades de pointes, cardiac arrest).
procarbazine	1	1	2	May result in CNS toxicity or serotonin syndrome (hypertension, hyperthermia, myoclonus, mental status changes).
procyclidine	1	3	2	May result in increased risk of anticholinergic effects (dry mouth, sedation, mydriasis).
propafenone	1	3	2	May result in increased risk of propafenone toxicity (cardiac arrhythmia).
protriptyline	2	3	2	May result in protriptyline toxicity (dry mouth, sedation, urinary retention).
quinidine	1	3	2	May result in elevated paroxetine plasma concentrations and possible paroxetine toxicity (nausea, dry mouth, somnolence, headache).
risperidone	2	3	2	May result in increased risk of risperidone adverse effects such as serotonin syndrome (hypertension, hyperthermia, myoclonus, mental status changes), extrapyramidal effects, and cardiotoxicity (QT prolongation, torsades de pointes, cardiac arrest) due to increased plasma risperidone levels.
ritonavir	0	3	2	May result in decreased paroxetine plasma levels.
rizatriptan	2	2	2	May result in increased risk of serotonin syndrome.

sibutramine	1	2	2	May result in increased risk of serotonin syndrome (hypertension, hyperthermia, myoclonus, mental status changes).
St. John's wort	1	2	2	May result in increased risk of serotonin syndrome (hypertension, hyperthermia, myoclonus, mental status changes).
sumatriptan	2	2	2	May result in increased risk of serotonin syndrome.
thioridazine	1	1	2	May result in increased risk of thioridazine toxicity, cardiotoxicity (QT prolongation, torsades de pointes, cardiac arrest).
toloxatone	1	1	2	May result in CNS toxicity or serotonin syndrome (hypertension, hyperthermia, myoclonus, mental status changes).
trazodone	1	2	2	May result in serotonin syndrome (hypertension, hyperthermia, myoclonus, mental status changes).
trimipramine	2	3	2	May result in trimipramine toxicity (dry mouth, sedation, urinary retention).
tryptophan	2	2	2	May result in serotonin syndrome (hypertension, hyperthermia, myoclonus, mental status changes).
warfarin	2	3	2	May result in increased risk of bleeding.
zolmitriptan	2	2	2	May result in serotonin syndrome.

PENICILLIN V

Tetracyclines (*minocycline, oxytetracycline, rolitetracycline, tetracycline*)	2	3	2	May result in decreased antibacterial effectiveness.

PHENOBARBITAL

acenocoumarol	2	2	2	May result in decreased anticoagulant effectiveness.
amprenavir	2	3	2	May result in reduced amprenavir efficacy.
betamethasone	2	3	2	May result in decreased betamethasone effectiveness.
bexarotene	0	3	2	May result in decreased plasma levels of bexarotene.
BZDs (*adinazolam, alprazolam, bromazepam, brotizolam, chlordiazepoxide, clobazam, clonazepam, clorazepate, diazepam, estazolam, flunitrazepam, flurazepam, halazepam, ketazolam, lorazepam, lormetazepam, lormetazepam, medazepam, midazolam, nitrazepam, nordazepam, oxazepam, prazepam, temazepam, triazolam*)	0	2	2	May result in additive respiratory depression.
cannabis	1	3	2	May result in increased CNS depression.
chlorpromazine	1	3	2	May result in decreased chlorpromazine effectiveness.

clozapine	2	3	2	May result in decreased clozapine plasma levels associated with marked worsening of psychosis.
Contraceptives, Combination (*ethinyl estradiol, etonogestrel, levonorgestrel, mestranol, norelgestromin, norethindrone, norgestrel*)	2	3	2	May result in decreased plasma concentrations of estrogens and in contraceptive effectiveness.
cortisone	2	3	2	May result in decreased cortisone effectiveness.
delavirdine	2	2	2	May result in decreased trough plasma delavirdine concentrations.
dexamethasone	2	3	2	May result in decreased dexamethasone effectiveness.
dicumarol	2	2	2	May result in decreased anticoagulant effectiveness.
digitoxin	2	3	2	May result in decreased digitoxin levels.
ethosuximide	2	3	2	May result in decreased ethosuximide serum concentrations.
felodipine	2	3	2	May result in decreased felodipine effectiveness.
fosamprenavir	2	3	2	May result in decreased amprenavir serum concentrations and reduced fosamprenavir efficacy.
ginkgo	2	3	2	May result in decreased anticonvulsant effectiveness.
granisetron	2	3	2	May result in increased plasma clearance of granisetron.
griseofulvin	1	3	2	May result in decreased effectiveness of griseofulvin.

ONSET: 0 - NOT SPECIFIED, 1 - RAPID, 2 - DELAYED   SEVERITY: 1 - CONTRAINDICATED, 2 - MAJOR, 3 - MODERATE

irinotecan	0	2	2	May result in substantially decreased exposure to irinotecan and its active metabolite SN-38 and may decrease irinotecan efficacy.
itraconazole	2	3	2	May result in loss of itraconazole efficacy.
lamotrigine	2	3	2	May result in reduced lamotrigine efficacy, loss of seizure control.
leucovorin	2	3	2	May result in decreased efficacy of phenobarbital.
levomethadyl	2	3	2	May result in increased risk of cardiotoxicity (QT prolongation, torsades de pointes).
lopinavir	2	2	2	May result in decreased lopinavir exposure.
methoxyflurane	1	2	2	May result in nephrotoxicity.
methylprednisolone	2	3	2	May result in decreased methylprednisolone effectiveness.
metoprolol	2	3	2	May result in decreased metoprolol effectiveness.
nimodipine	2	3	2	May result in decreased nimodipine effectiveness.
Opioid Analgesics (*alfentanil, anileridine, codeine, fentanyl, hydrocodone, hydromorphone, levorphanol, meperidine, morphine, morphine sulfate liposome, oxycodone, oxymorphone, propoxyphene, remifentanil, sufentanil*)	0	2	2	May result in additive respiratory depression.

Drug	Onset	Severity		Description
oxcarbazepine	2	3	2	May result in decreased concentration of the active 10-monohydroxy metabolite of oxcarbazepine and potential loss of oxcarbazepine efficacy.
phenprocoumon	2	2	2	May result in decreased anticoagulant effectiveness.
prednisone	2	3	2	May result in decreased therapeutic effect of prednisone.
quetiapine	0	2	2	May result in decreased serum quetiapine concentrations.
quinidine	2	3	2	May result in decreased quinidine effectiveness.
risperidone	2	3	2	May result in decreased plasma concentrations of risperidone and the active metabolite 9-hydroxyrisperidone.
saquinavir	1	3	2	May result in reduced saquinavir effectiveness.
telithromycin	0	3	2	May result in subtherapeutic telithromycin concentrations.
teniposide	2	2	2	May result in increased teniposide clearance.
theophylline	2	3	2	May result in decreased theophylline effectiveness.
thioridazine	1	3	2	May result in decreased phenobarbital or thioridazine effectiveness.
tiagabine	2	3	2	May result in decreased tiagabine efficacy.
topiramate	2	3	2	May result in decreased serum concentrations of topiramate.
valproic acid	2	3	2	May result in phenobarbital toxicity or decreased valproic acid effectiveness.

ONSET: 0 - NOT SPECIFIED 1 - RAPID 2 - DELAYED   SEVERITY: 1 - CONTRAINDICATED 2 - MAJOR 3 - MODERATE

verapamil	2	3	2	May result in decreased verapamil effectiveness.
warfarin	2	3	1	May result in decreased anticoagulant effectiveness.

PHENTERMINE

fenfluramine	2	2	1	May result in increased risk of pulmonary hypertension and valvular heart disease.
MAOIs (*clorgyline, iproniazide, isocarboxazid, moclobemide, nialamide, pargyline, phenelzine, procarbazine, selegiline, toloxatone, tranylcypromine*)	1	1	2	May result in hypertensive crisis (headache, hyperpyrexia, hypertension).

PHENYTOIN

acetaminophen	2	3	2	May result in decreased acetaminophen effectiveness and an increased risk of hepatotoxicity.
acetazolamide	2	3	2	May result in increased risk of osteomalacia.
acyclovir	2	3	2	May result in decreased phenytoin plasma concentrations and potential increased seizure activity.
amiodarone	2	3	2	May result in increased risk of phenytoin toxicity (ataxia, hyperreflexia, nystagmus, tremor) and/or decreased amiodarone concentrations.
amitriptyline	2	3	2	May result in increased risk of phenytoin toxicity (ataxia, hyperreflexia, nystagmus, tremor).
amprenavir	2	3	2	May result in reduced amprenavir efficacy.

Drug	Onset	Severity		Effect
apazone	2	2	2	May result in increased risk of phenytoin toxicity.
aprepitant	2	3	2	May result in reduced efficacy and serum concentrations of aprepitant and phenytoin.
atorvastatin	2	3	2	May result in loss of atorvastatin efficacy.
beclamide	2	2	2	May result in leukopenia.
betamethasone	2	3	2	May result in decreased betamethasone effectiveness.
bexarotene	0	3	2	May result in decreased plasma levels of bexarotene.
bleomycin	1	3	2	May result in decreased phenytoin effectiveness.
busulfan	2	3	2	May result in decreased plasma concentrations of busulfan.
capecitabine	2	3	2	May result in increased phenytoin levels and associated phenytoin toxicity.
carbamazepine	2	3	2	May result in increased phenytoin concentrations and decreased carbamazepine concentrations.
carboplatin	1	3	2	May result in decreased phenytoin effectiveness.
caspofungin	2	3	2	May result in reduced caspofungin plasma levels.
chloramphenicol	2	3	2	May result in increased risk of phenytoin toxicity (ataxia, hyperreflexia, nystagmus, tremor).
cimetidine	2	3	2	May result in increased risk of phenytoin toxicity (ataxia, hyperreflexia, nystagmus, tremor).

ONSET: 0 - NOT SPECIFIED 1 - RAPID 2 - DELAYED   SEVERITY: 1 - CONTRAINDICATED 2 - MAJOR 3 - MODERATE

ciprofloxacin	2	3	2	May result in increased or decreased phenytoin levels.
cisplatin	1	3	2	May result in decreased phenytoin plasma concentrations.
clarithromycin	2	3	2	May result in increased risk of phenytoin toxicity (ataxia, hyperreflexia, nystagmus, tremor).
clobazam	2	3	2	May result in increased risk of phenytoin toxicity (ataxia, hyperreflexia, nystagmus, tremor).
clofazimine	2	3	2	May result in reduced phenytoin serum concentrations and loss of phenytoin efficacy.
clopidogrel	2	3	2	May result in increased risk of phenytoin toxicity (ataxia, hyperreflexia, nystagmus, tremor).
clozapine	2	3	2	May result in decreased clozapine plasma levels associated with marked worsening of psychosis.
Contraceptives, Combination (*ethinyl estradiol, etonogestrel, levonorgestrel, mestranol, norelgestromin, norethindrone, norgestrel*)	2	3	2	May result in decreased contraceptive effectiveness.
cortisone	2	3	2	May result in decreased cortisone effectiveness.
cyclosporine	2	3	2	May result in reduced cyclosporine serum levels and potentially increased risk of organ rejection.
delavirdine	2	2	2	May result in decreased trough plasma delavirdine concentrations.

dexamethasone	2	3	1	May result in decreased dexamethasone effectiveness.
diazepam	2	3	2	May result in alterations in serum phenytoin concentrations.
dicumarol	2	3	2	May result in transient increased risk of bleeding when beginning phenytoin therapy, decreased anticoagulant efficacy during chronic therapy, and/or phenytoin toxicity.
digitoxin	2	3	2	May result in decreased serum digitoxin concentrations.
diltiazem	2	3	2	May result in increased risk of phenytoin toxicity (ataxia, hyperreflexia, nystagmus, tremor).
disopyramide	2	3	2	May result in decreased disopyramide effectiveness.
disulfiram	2	3	2	May result in increased risk of phenytoin toxicity (ataxia, hyperreflexia, nystagmus, tremors).
doxepin	2	3	2	May result in increased risk of phenytoin toxicity (ataxia, hyperreflexia, nystagmus, tremor).
doxorubicin hydrochloride	2	3	2	May result in decreased phenytoin effectiveness.
enteral nutrition	1	3	2	May result in decreased serum phenytoin levels and subsequently reduced therapeutic response to phenytoin.
ethanol	1	3	2	May result in decreased phenytoin serum concentrations, increased seizure potential, and additive CNS depressant effects.

ONSET: 0 — NOT SPECIFIED, 1 — RAPID, 2 — DELAYED   SEVERITY: 1 — CONTRAINDICATED, 2 — MAJOR, 3 — MODERATE

ethosuximide	2	3	2	May result in decreased ethosuximide serum concentrations.
felbamate	2	3	2	May result in increased risk of phenytoin toxicity (ataxia, hyperreflexia, nystagmus, tremors); decreased felbamate levels.
fentanyl	2	3	2	May result in decreased plasma concentrations of fentanyl.
fluconazole	2	3	2	May result in increased risk of phenytoin toxicity (ataxia, hyperreflexia, nystagmus, tremors).
fludrocortisone	2	3	2	May result in decreased fludrocortisone effectiveness.
fluorouracil	0	3	2	May result in increased serum phenytoin levels and phenytoin toxicity (ataxia, hyperreflexia, nystagmus, tremor).
fluoxetine	2	3	2	May result in increased risk of phenytoin toxicity (ataxia, hyperreflexia, nystagmus, tremor).
fluvoxamine	2	3	2	May result in increased risk of phenytoin toxicity (ataxia, hyperreflexia, nystagmus, tremors).
folic acid	2	3	2	May result in decreased phenytoin effectiveness.
fosamprenavir	2	3	2	May result in decreased amprenavir serum concentrations and reduced fosamprenavir efficacy.
gefitinib	0	3	2	May result in decreased plasma gefitinib concentrations.
ginkgo	2	3	2	May result in decreased anticonvulsant effectiveness.

ibuprofen	2	3	2	May result in increased risk of phenytoin toxicity (ataxia, hyperreflexia, nystagmus, tremor), especially in renally impaired patients.
imatinib	2	2	2	May result in decreased plasma concentrations of imatinib.
imipramine	2	3	2	May result in increased risk of phenytoin toxicity (ataxia, hyperreflexia, nystagmus, tremors).
irinotecan	0	2	2	May result in decreased exposure to irinotecan and its active metabolite (SN-38) and may decrease chemotherapeutic efficacy.
isoniazid	2	3	2	May result in increased risk of phenytoin toxicity (ataxia, hyperreflexia, nystagmus, tremor).
itraconazole	2	3	2	May result in decreased serum itraconazole concentrations and loss of antimycotic efficacy.
levodopa	2	3	2	May result in decreased levodopa effectiveness.
levomethadyl	2	3	2	May result in increased risk of cardiotoxicity (QT prolongation, torsades de pointes).
levothyroxine	2	3	2	May result in decreased levothyroxine effectiveness.
lidocaine	1	2	2	May result in additive cardiac depressive effects; decreased lidocaine serum concentrations.
lopinavir	2	2	2	May result in decreased lopinavir exposure.

ONSET: 0 = SPECIFIED, 1 = RAPID, 2 = DELAYED   SEVERITY: 1 = CONTRAINDICATED, 2 = MAJOR, 3 = MODERATE

methotrexate	1	2	2	May result in decreased phenytoin effectiveness and an increased risk of methotrexate toxicity (myelotoxicity, pancytopenia, megaloblastic anemia).
methoxsalen	2	3	2	May result in decreased methoxsalen effectiveness.
methsuximide	2	3	2	May result in increased risk of phenytoin toxicity (ataxia, hyperreflexia, nystagmus, tremor).
miconazole	2	3	2	May result in increased risk of phenytoin toxicity (ataxia, hyperreflexia, nystagmus, tremor).
midazolam	1	3	2	May result in decreased efficacy of midazolam.
nafimidone	1	3	2	May result in increased risk of phenytoin toxicity (ataxia, hyperreflexia, nystagmus, tremor).
nelfinavir	2	3	2	May result in reduced phenytoin efficacy.
nifedipine	2	3	2	May result in increased risk of phenytoin toxicity (ataxia, hyperreflexia, nystagmus, tremor).
nilutamide	2	3	2	May result in increased risk of phenytoin toxicity (ataxia, hyperreflexia, nystagmus, or tremor).
nisoldipine	2	3	2	May result in decreased nisoldipine plasma concentrations.
oxcarbazepine	2	3	2	May result in increased risk of phenytoin toxicity (ataxia, hyperreflexia, nystagmus, tremor).
paclitaxel	2	3	2	May result in loss of paclitaxel efficacy.

	Onset	Severity		Description
pancuronium	1	3	2	May result in decreased or increased pancuronium effectiveness.
paroxetine	2	3	2	May result in reduced phenytoin efficacy; reduced paroxetine efficacy.
phenprocoumon	2	3	2	May result in transient increased risk of bleeding when beginning phenytoin therapy, decreased anticoagulant effectiveness during chronic therapy, phenytoin toxicity.
piperine	1	3	2	May result in increased bioavailability of phenytoin (ataxia, hyperreflexia, nystagmus, tremor).
posaconazole	0	2	2	May result in decreased posaconazole concentration and increased phenytoin concentration.
praziquantel	2	3	2	May result in decreased praziquantel effectiveness.
prednisolone	2	3	2	May result in decreased prednisolone effectiveness.
prednisone	2	3	2	May result in decreased prednisone effectiveness.
progabide	2	3	2	May result in increased risk of phenytoin toxicity (nausea, vomiting, palpitations, seizures).
quetiapine	2	3	1	May result in decreased quetiapine efficacy.
quinidine	2	3	2	May result in decreased quinidine effectiveness.
remacemide	2	3	2	May result in reduced remacemide exposure and increased phenytoin exposure.

ONSET: 0 - NOT SPECIFIED, 1 - RAPID, 2 - DELAYED   SEVERITY: 1 - CONTRAINDICATED, 2 - MAJOR, 3 - MODERATE

rifampin	2	3	2	May result in decreased phenytoin effectiveness.
rifapentine	2	3	2	May result in decreased anticonvulsant effectiveness.
risperidone	2	3	2	May result in decreased plasma concentrations of risperidone and the active metabolite 9-hydroxyrisperidone.
ritonavir	2	3	2	May result in decreases in phenytoin serum concentrations.
sabeluzole	2	3	2	May result in reduced sabeluzole efficacy.
saquinavir	1	3	2	May result in reduced saquinavir effectiveness.
sertraline	2	3	2	May result in increased risk of phenytoin toxicity (ataxia, hyperreflexia, nystagmus, tremor).
shankhapulshpi	2	3	2	May result in decreased plasma levels and effectiveness of phenytoin.
simvastatin	2	3	2	May result in loss of simvastatin efficacy.
sirolimus	2	3	2	May result in loss of sirolimus efficacy.
St. John's wort	2	2	2	May result in reduced phenytoin effectiveness.
sulfamethizole	2	3	2	May result in increased risk of phenytoin toxicity (ataxia, hyperreflexia, nystagmus, tremor).
sulfaphenazole	2	3	2	May result in increased risk of phenytoin toxicity (ataxia, hyperreflexia, nystagmus, tremors).
sulthiame	2	3	2	May result in increased risk of phenytoin toxicity (ataxia, hyperreflexia, nystagmus, tremor).

tacrolimus	2	2	2	May result in decreased tacrolimus efficacy or increased serum phenytoin concentrations.
telithromycin	0	3	2	May result in subtherapeutic telithromycin concentrations and/or elevation of serum levels of phenytoin.
tenidap	2	3	2	May result in increased unbound phenytoin levels.
theophylline	2	3	2	May result in decreased theophylline effectiveness.
tiagabine	2	3	2	May result in decreased tiagabine efficacy.
ticlopidine	2	3	2	May result in increased risk of phenytoin toxicity (ataxia, hyperreflexia, nystagmus, tremor).
ticrynafen	2	3	2	May result in increased risk of phenytoin toxicity (ataxia, hyperreflexia, nystagmus, tremor).
tirilazad	2	3	2	May result in decreased tirilazad efficacy.
tizanidine	2	3	2	May result in increased risk of phenytoin toxicity (ataxia, hyperreflexia, nystagmus, tremor).
tolbutamide	2	3	2	May result in increased risk of phenytoin toxicity (ataxia, hyperreflexia, nystagmus, tremor).
topiramate	2	3	2	May result in altered topiramate or phenytoin concentrations.
trazodone	0	3	2	May result in increased phenytoin serum concentrations and an increased risk of phenytoin toxicity (ataxia, hyperreflexia, nystagmus, tremor).

ONSET: 0 = NOT SPECIFIED, 1 = RAPID, 2 = DELAYED   SEVERITY: 1 = CONTRAINDICATED, 2 = MAJOR, 3 = MODERATE

triamcinolone	2	3	2	May result in decreased triamcinolone effectiveness.
trimethoprim	2	3	2	May result in increased risk of phenytoin toxicity (ataxia, hyperreflexia, nystagmus, tremors).
tubocurarine	1	3	2	May result in decreased or increased tubocurarine effectiveness.
valproic acid	2	3	2	May result in altered valproate levels or altered phenytoin levels.
vecuronium	1	3	2	May result in decreased or increased vecuronium effectiveness.
verapamil	2	3	2	May result in decreased verapamil effectiveness.
viloxazine	2	3	2	May result in increased risk of phenytoin toxicity (ataxia, hyperreflexia, nystagmus, tremor).
voriconazole	0	2	1	May result in increased plasma phenytoin concentrations and decreased plasma voriconazole concentrations.
PIOGLITAZONE				
atorvastatin	2	3	2	May result in reduced pioglitazone bioavailability and increased risk of hyperglycemia.
bitter melon	1	3	2	May result in increased risk of hypoglycemia.
ethinyl estradiol	2	3	2	May result in loss of contraceptive efficacy.
fenugreek	1	3	2	May result in increased risk of hypoglycemia.

gemfibrozil	2	3	2	May result in increased pioglitazone concentrations and potentially increased risk of hypoglycemia.
glucomannan	1	3	2	May result in increased risk of hypoglycemia.
guar gum	1	3	2	May result in increased risk of hypoglycemia.
ketoconazole	2	3	2	May result in increased pioglitazone serum concentrations and increased risk of hypoglycemia (CNS depression, seizures, diaphoresis, tachypnea, tachycardia, hypothermia).
levonorgestrel	2	3	2	May result in loss of contraceptive efficacy.
mestranol	2	3	2	May result in loss of contraceptive efficacy.
norethindrone	2	3	2	May result in loss of contraceptive efficacy.
norgestrel	2	3	2	May result in loss of contraceptive efficacy.
psyllium	1	3	2	May result in increased risk of hypoglycemia.
rifampin	2	3	1	May result in decreased pioglitazone exposure.
St. John's wort	1	3	2	May result in hypoglycemia.
topiramate	2	3	2	May result in decreased pioglitazone exposure.
POTASSIUM				
amiloride	2	2	2	May result in hyperkalemia.
benazepril	2	2	2	May result in hyperkalemia.
canrenoate	2	2	2	May result in hyperkalemia.

ONSET: 0 - NOT SPECIFIED 1 - RAPID 2 - DELAYED   SEVERITY: 1 - CONTRAINDICATED 2 - MAJOR 3 - MODERATE

captopril	2	2	2	May result in hyperkalemia.
delapril	2	2	2	May result in hyperkalemia.
enalapril maleate	2	2	2	May result in hyperkalemia.
enalaprilat	2	2	2	May result in hyperkalemia.
fosinopril	2	2	2	May result in hyperkalemia.
imidapril	2	2	2	May result in hyperkalemia.
indomethacin	2	2	2	May result in hyperkalemia.
licorice	2	3	2	May result in reduced effectiveness of potassium.
lisinopril	2	2	1	May result in hyperkalemia.
quinapril	2	2	2	May result in hyperkalemia.
ramipril	2	2	2	May result in hyperkalemia.
temocapril	2	2	2	May result in hyperkalemia.
trandolapril	2	2	2	May result in hyperkalemia.
PRAVASTATIN				
amprenavir	2	3	2	May result in increased risk of myopathy or rhabdomyolysis.
bezafibrate	2	2	2	May result in increased risk of myopathy or rhabdomyolysis.
ciprofibrate	2	2	2	May result in increased risk of myopathy or rhabdomyolysis.

cyclosporine	2	3	2	May result in increased risk of myopathy or rhabdomyolysis.
dalfopristin	2	2	2	May result in increased risk of myopathy or rhabdomyolysis.
darunavir	0	3	1	May result in increased exposure to pravastatin.
efavirenz	2	3	1	May result in decreased pravastatin plasma concentrations.
fenofibrate	0	2	2	May result in increased risk of myopathy or rhabdomyolysis.
gemfibrozil	2	2	2	May result in increased risk of myopathy or rhabdomyolysis.
nefazodone	2	3	2	May result in increased risk of myopathy or rhabdomyolysis.
nelfinavir	2	3	1	May result in decreased pravastatin plasma concentration.
oat bran	2	3	2	May result in reduced effectiveness of HMG CoA reductase inhibitors.
pectin	2	3	2	May result in reduced effectiveness of HMG CoA reductase inhibitors.
quinupristin	2	2	2	May result in increased risk of myopathy or rhabdomyolysis.

ONSET: 0 - NOT SPECIFIED 1 - RAPID 2 - DELAYED   SEVERITY: 1 - CONTRAINDICATED 2 - MAJOR 3 - MODERATE

PREDNISOLONE

Drug				Effect
alcuronium	2	3	2	May result in decreased alcuronium effectiveness; prolonged muscle weakness and myopathy.
amobarbital	2	3	2	May result in decreased therapeutic effect of prednisolone.
aspirin	2	3	2	May result in increased risk of gastrointestinal ulceration and subtherapeutic aspirin serum concentrations.
atracurium	2	3	2	May result in decreased atracurium effectiveness; prolonged muscle weakness and myopathy.
Contraceptives, Combination (*desogestrel, drospirenone, ethinyl estradiol, ethynodiol diacetate, levonorgestrel, mestranol, norelgestromin, norethindrone, norgestimate, norgestrel*)	2	3	1	May result in increased risk of corticosteroid side effects (neuropsychiatric reactions, fluid and electrolyte disturbances, hypertension, hyperglycemia).
FLQs (*alatrofloxacin, balofloxacin, cinoxacin, ciprofloxacin, clinafloxacin, enoxacin, fleroxacin, flumequine, gemifloxacin, grepafloxacin, levofloxacin, lomefloxacin, moxifloxacin, norfloxacin, ofloxacin, pefloxacin, prulifloxacin, rosoxacin, rufloxacin, sparfloxacin, temafloxacin, tosufloxacin, trovafloxacin*)	2	3	1	May result in increased risk for tendon rupture.
fosphenytoin	2	3	2	May result in decreased prednisolone effectiveness.

Drug	Onset	Severity		Description
gallamine	2	3	2	May result in decreased gallamine effectiveness; prolonged muscle weakness and myopathy.
hexafluorenium	2	3	2	May result in decreased hexafluorenium bromide effectiveness; prolonged muscle weakness and myopathy.
itraconazole	2	3	2	May result in increased corticosteroid plasma concentrations and an increased risk of corticosteroid side effects (myopathy, glucose intolerance, Cushing's syndrome).
licorice	2	3	2	May result in increased risk of corticosteroid adverse effects.
metocurine	2	3	2	May result in decreased metocurine effectiveness; prolonged muscle weakness and myopathy.
phenytoin	2	3	2	May result in decreased prednisolone effectiveness.
primidone	2	3	2	May result in decreased prednisolone effectiveness.
quetiapine	0	2	2	May result in decreased serum quetiapine concentrations.
rifampin	2	3	2	May result in decreased prednisolone effectiveness.
rotavirus vaccine, live	2	1	1	May result in increased risk of infection by the live vaccine.
saiboku-to	2	3	2	May result in enhanced and prolonged effect of corticosteroids.
vecuronium	2	3	2	May result in decreased vecuronium effectiveness; prolonged muscle weakness and myopathy.

ONSET: 0 = NOT SPECIFIED 1 = RAPID 2 = DELAYED   SEVERITY: 1 = CONTRAINDICATED 2 = MAJOR 3 = MODERATE

PREDNISONE

alcuronium	2	3	2	May result in decreased alcuronium effectiveness; prolonged muscle weakness and myopathy.
alfalfa	2	3	1	May result in reduced prednisone effectiveness.
amobarbital	2	3	2	May result in decreased therapeutic effect of prednisone.
aprobarbital	2	3	2	May result in decreased therapeutic effect of prednisone.
aspirin	2	3	2	May result in increased risk of gastrointestinal ulceration and subtherapeutic aspirin serum concentrations.
atracurium	2	3	2	May result in decreased atracurium effectiveness; prolonged muscle weakness and myopathy.
butabarbital	2	3	2	May result in decreased therapeutic effect of prednisone.
butalbital	2	3	2	May result in decreased therapeutic effect of prednisone.
clarithromycin	2	3	2	May result in increased risk of psychotic symptoms.
fluconazole	2	3	2	May result in decreased metabolic degradation of prednisone and increased prednisone efficacy.
fosphenytoin	2	3	2	May result in decreased prednisone effectiveness.
gallamine	2	3	2	May result in decreased gallamine effectiveness; prolonged muscle weakness and myopathy.
gatifloxacin	2	2	2	May result in increased blood glucose and risk of hyperglycemia.

hexafluorenium	2	3	2	May result in decreased hexafluorenium bromide effectiveness; prolonged muscle weakness and myopathy.
itraconazole	2	3	2	May result in increased corticosteroid plasma concentrations and an increased risk of corticosteroid side effects (myopathy, glucose intolerance, Cushing's syndrome).
ketoconazole	2	3	2	May result in increased risk of corticosteroid side effects (neuropsychiatric reactions, fluid and electrolyte disturbances, hypertension, hyperglycemia).
licorice	2	3	2	May result in increased risk of corticosteroid adverse effects.
mephobarbital	2	3	2	May result in decreased therapeutic effect of prednisone.
metocurine	2	3	2	May result in decreased metocurine effectiveness; prolonged muscle weakness and myopathy.
montelukast	2	3	2	May result in severe peripheral edema.
pancuronium	2	3	2	May result in decreased pancuronium effectiveness; prolonged muscle weakness and myopathy.
phenobarbital	2	3	2	May result in decreased therapeutic effect of prednisone.
phenytoin	2	3	2	May result in decreased prednisone effectiveness.
primidone	2	3	2	May result in decreased therapeutic effect of prednisone.
quetiapine	0	2	2	May result in decreased serum quetiapine concentrations.
rifampin	2	3	2	May result in decreased prednisone effectiveness.

ONSET: 0 - NOT SPECIFIED 1 - RAPID 2 - DELAYED   SEVERITY: 1 - CONTRAINDICATED 2 - MAJOR 3 - MODERATE

rifapentine	2	3	2	May result in decreased corticosteroid effectiveness.
ritonavir	2	3	2	May result in increased prednisone serum concentrations.
rotavirus vaccine, live	2	1	1	May result in increased risk of infection by the live vaccine.
saiboku-to	2	3	2	May result in enhanced and prolonged effect of corticosteroids.
secobarbital	2	3	2	May result in decreased therapeutic effect of prednisone.
vecuronium	2	3	2	May result in decreased vecuronium effectiveness; prolonged muscle weakness and myopathy.
PROMETHAZINE				
belladonna	1	3	2	May result in increased manic, agitated reactions, or enhanced anticholinergic effects resulting in cardiorespiratory failure, especially in cases of belladonna overdose.
belladonna alkaloids	1	3	2	May result in increased manic, agitated reactions, or enhanced anticholinergic effects resulting in cardiorespiratory failure, especially in cases of belladonna overdose.
betel nut	2	3	2	May result in increased extrapyramidal side effects of phenothiazines.
cisapride	1	1	2	May result in cardiotoxicity (QT prolongation, torsades de pointes, cardiac arrest).

duloxetine	0	3	2	May result in increased phenothiazine serum concentrations and potential toxicity (sedation, confusion, cardiac arrhythmias, orthostatic hypotension, hyperthermia, extrapyramidal effects).
evening primrose	2	3	2	May result in increased risk of seizures.
gatifloxacin	1	2	2	May result in increased risk of cardiotoxicity (QT prolongation, torsades de pointes, cardiac arrest).
grepafloxacin	2	1	2	May result in increased risk of cardiotoxicity (QT prolongation, torsades de pointes, cardiac arrest).
lithium	2	2	2	May result in weakness, dyskinesias, increased extrapyramidal symptoms, encephalopathy, and brain damage.
meperidine	1	3	2	May result in increased CNS and respiratory depression.
phenylalanine	1	3	2	May result in increased incidence of tardive dyskinesia.
procarbazine	2	2	2	May result in CNS depression.
sparfloxacin	2	1	2	May result in prolongation of the QTc interval and/or torsades de pointes.
urine chorionic gonadotropin measurement	1	3	2	May result in falsely positive or negative pregnancy test results due to interference based on immunological reactions between human chorionic gonadotropin (HCG) and anti-HCG.

ONSET: 0 - NOT SPECIFIED, 1 - RAPID, 2 - DELAYED   SEVERITY: 1 - CONTRAINDICATED, 2 - MAJOR, 3 - MODERATE

PROPOXYPHENE

Drug				Effect
Barbiturates (amobarbital, aprobarbital, butabarbital, butalbital, mephobarbital, methohexital, pentobarbital, phenobarbital, primidone, secobarbital, thiopental)	0	2	2	May result in additive respiratory depression.
BZDs (adinazolam, alprazolam, bromazepam, brotizolam, chlordiazepoxide, clobazam, clonazepam, clorazepate, diazepam, estazolam, flunitrazepam, flurazepam, halazepam, ketazolam, lorazepam, lormetazepam, lormetazepam, medazepam, midazolam, nitrazepam, nordazepam, oxazepam, prazepam, temazepam, triazolam)	0	2	2	May result in additive respiratory depression.
carbamazepine	2	2	2	May result in increased risk of carbamazepine toxicity (ataxia, nystagmus, diplopia, headache, vomiting, apnea, seizures, coma).
doxepin	2	3	2	May result in doxepin toxicity (sedation, lethargy, dry mouth, urinary retention).
metoprolol	1	3	2	May result in increased risk of hypotension and bradycardia.

Muscle Relaxants, Centrally Acting (*carisoprodol, chlorzoxazone, dantrolene, mephenesin, meprobamate, metaxalone, methocarbamol*)	0	2	2	May result in additive respiratory depression.
naltrexone	1	1	2	May result in precipitation of opioid withdrawal symptoms; decreased opioid effectiveness.
Opioid Agonists/Antagonists (*buprenorphine, butorphanol, dezocine, nalbuphine, pentazocine*)	0	2	2	May result in additive respiratory depression.
propranolol	1	3	2	May result in increased risk of hypotension and bradycardia.
warfarin	2	3	2	May result in increased risk of bleeding.
PSEUDOEPHEDRINE				
clorgyline	1	1	1	May result in severe hypertension, hyperpyrexia, headache.
guanethidine	1	2	2	May result in loss of blood pressure control and possibly result in the development of cardiac arrhythmias.
iproniazid	1	1	2	May result in severe hypertension, hyperpyrexia, headache.
linezolid	1	2	2	May result in increased blood pressure.
methyldopa	1	2	2	May result in loss of blood pressure control and possibly hypertensive urgency.
moclobemide	1	1	2	May result in severe hypertension, hyperpyrexia, headache.

ONSET: 0 = NOT SPECIFIED 1 = RAPID 2 = DELAYED   SEVERITY: 1 = CONTRAINDICATED 2 = MAJOR 3 = MODERATE

nialamide	1	1	2	May result in hypertensive crisis (headache, hyperpyrexia, hypertension).
pargyline	1	1	2	May result in hypertensive crisis (headache, hyperpyrexia, hypertension).
procarbazine	1	1	2	May result in severe hypertension, hyperpyrexia, headache.
toloxatone	1	1	2	May result in severe hypertension, hyperpyrexia, headache.
QUETIAPINE				
Antiarrhythmic Agents, Class IA (ajmaline, disopyramide, moricizine, pirmenol, prajmaline, procainamide, quinidine, recainam)	0	2	2	May result in increased risk of cardiotoxicity (QT prolongation, torsades de pointes, cardiac arrest).
Barbiturates (amobarbital, aprobarbital, butabarbital, butalbital, mephobarbital, methohexital, pentobarbital, phenobarbital, primidone, secobarbital, thiopental)	0	2	2	May result in decreased serum quetiapine concentrations.
erythromycin	2	2	2	May result in increased quetiapine serum concentrations; an increased risk of cardiotoxicity (QT prolongation, torsades de pointes, cardiac arrest).
ethanol	1	3	2	May result in potentiation of the cognitive and motor effects of alcohol.

fluconazole	2	2	2	May result in increased quetiapine serum concentrations; an increased risk of cardiotoxicity (QT prolongation, torsades de pointes, cardiac arrest).
fosphenytoin	2	3	2	May result in decreased quetiapine efficacy.
Glucocorticoids (*betamethasone, cortisone, deflazacort, dexamethasone, hydrocortisone, methylprednisolone, paramethasone, prednisolone, prednisone, triamcinolone*)	0	2	2	May result in decreased serum quetiapine concentrations.
haloperidol	0	2	2	May result in increased risk of cardiotoxicity (QT prolongation, torsades de pointes, cardiac arrest).
itraconazole	2	3	2	May result in increased quetiapine serum concentrations.
ketoconazole	2	3	2	May result in increased quetiapine serum concentrations.
phenytoin	2	3	1	May result in decreased quetiapine efficacy.
rifampin	0	2	2	May result in decreased serum quetiapine concentrations.
risperidone	0	2	2	May result in increased risk of cardiotoxicity (QT prolongation, torsades de pointes, cardiac arrest).
warfarin	2	3	2	May result in potentiation of anticoagulant effects.
QUINAPRIL				
aliskiren	0	3	2	May result in hyperkalemia.

ONSET: 0 = NOT SPECIFIED, 1 = RAPID, 2 = DELAYED   SEVERITY: 1 = CONTRAINDIC[A]TED, 2 = MAJOR, 3 = MODERATE

	2	3	2	
bupivacaine	2	3	2	May result in bradycardia and hypotension with loss of consciousness.
capsaicin	1	3	2	May result in increased risk of cough.
lithium	2	3	2	May result in lithium toxicity (weakness, tremor, excessive thirst, confusion) and/or nephrotoxicity.
Loop Diuretics (*azosemide, bumetanide, ethacrynic acid, furosemide, piretanide, torsemide*)	1	3	2	May result in postural hypotension (first dose).
nesiritide	2	3	2	May result in increased symptomatic hypotension.
NSAIDs (*aceclofenac, acemetacin, alclofenac, apazone, aspirin, benoxaprofen, bromfenac, bufexamac, carprofen, celecoxib, clometacin, clonixin, dexketoprofen, diclofenac, diflunisal, dipyrone, dofetilide, droxicam, etodolac, etofenamate, felbinac, fenbufen, fenoprofen, fentiazac, floctafenine, flufenamic acid, flurbiprofen, ibuprofen, indomethacin, indoprofen, isoxicam, ketoprofen, ketorolac, lornoxicam, meclofenamate, mefenamic acid, meloxicam, nabumetone, naproxen, niflumic acid, nimesulide, oxaprozin, oxyphenbutazone,*	2	3	2	May result in decreased antihypertensive and natriuretic effects.

phenylbutazone, pirazolac, piroxicam, pirprofen, propyphenazon, proquazone, rofecoxib, sulindac, suprofen, tenidap, tenoxicam, tiaprofenic acid, ticrynafen, tolmetin, zomepirac)				
potassium	2	2	2	May result in hyperkalemia.
Potassium-Sparing Diuretics (amiloride, canrenoate, eplerenone, spironolactone, triamterene, torsemide)	2	2	2	May result in hyperkalemia.
Thiazide Diuretics (bemetizide, bendroflumethiazide, benzthiazide, buthiazide, chlorthiazide, chlorthalidone, clopamide, cyclopenthiazide, cyclothiazide, HCTZ, hydroflumethiazide, indapamide, methyclothiazide, metolazone, polythiazide, quinethazone, trichlormethiazide, xipamide)	1	3	2	May result in postural hypotension (first dose).
trimethoprim	2	3	2	May result in hyperkalemia.
QUININE				
cyclosporine	2	3	2	May result in decreased cyclosporine effectiveness.
digoxin	2	2	2	May result in digoxin toxicity (nausea, vomiting, cardiac arrhythmias).

ONSET: 0 – NOT SPECIFIED, 1 – RAPID, 2 – DELAYED   SEVERITY: 1 – CONTRAINDICATED, 2 – MAJOR, 3 – MODERATE

mefloquine	2	2	2	May result in increased risk of convulsions, electrocardiographic abnormalities, cardiac arrest, and decreased mefloquine efficacy.
rifapentine	2	3	2	May result in decreased quinine efficacy.
RABEPRAZOLE				
cranberry	1	3	2	May result in reduced effectiveness of proton pump inhibitors.
digoxin	2	3	2	May result in increased risk of digoxin toxicity (nausea, vomiting, arrhythmias).
itraconazole	2	3	2	May result in loss of itraconazole efficacy.
ketoconazole	1	3	2	May result in loss of ketoconazole efficacy.
RAMIPRIL				
aliskiren	0	3	2	May result in hyperkalemia.
bupivacaine	2	3	2	May result in bradycardia and hypotension with loss of consciousness.
capsaicin	1	3	2	May result in increased risk of cough.
Loop Diuretics (*azosemide, bumetanide, ethacrynic acid, furosemide, piretanide, torsemide*)	1	3	2	May result in postural hypotension (first dose).
nesiritide	2	3	2	May result in increased symptomatic hypotension.

potassium	2	2	2	May result in hyperkalemia.
Potassium-Sparing Diuretics (*amiloride, canrenoate, eplerenone, spironolactone, triamterene, torsemide*)	2	2	2	May result in hyperkalemia.
NSAIDs (*aceclofenac, acemetacin, alclofenac, apazone, aspirin, benoxaprofen, bromfenac, bufexamac, carprofen, celecoxib, clometacin, clonixin, dexketoprofen, diclofenac, diflunisal, dipyrone, dofetilide, droxicam, etodolac, etofenamate, felbinac, fenbufen, fenoprofen, fentiazac, floctafenine, flufenamic acid, flurbiprofen, ibuprofen, indomethacin, indoprofen, isoxicam, ketoprofen, ketorolac, lornoxicam, meclofenamate, mefenamic acid, meloxicam, nabumetone, naproxen, niflumic acid, nimesulide, oxaprozin, oxyphenbutazone, phenylbutazone, pirazolac, piroxicam, pirprofen, propyphenazon, proquazone, rofecoxib, sulindac, suprofen, tenidap, tenoxicam, tiaprofenic acid, ticrynafen, tolmetin, zomepirac*)	2	3	2	May result in decreased antihypertensive and natriuretic effects.

ONSET: 0 = NOT SPECIFIED 1 = RAPID 2 = DELAYED   SEVERITY: 1 = CONTRAINDICATED 2 = MAJOR 3 = MODERATE
EVIDENCE: 1 = EXCELLENT 2 = GOOD

INTERACTING DRUG	ONSET	SEVERITY	EVIDENCE	WARNING
Thiazide Diuretics (*bemetizide, bendroflumethiazide, benzthiazide, buthiazide, chlorthiazide, chlorthalidone, clopamide, cyclopenthiazide, cyclothiazide, HCTZ, hydroflumethiazide, indapamide, methyclothiazide, metolazone, polythiazide, quinethazone, trichlormethiazide, xipamide*)	1	3	2	May result in postural hypotension (first dose).

RANITIDINE

INTERACTING DRUG	ONSET	SEVERITY	EVIDENCE	WARNING
atazanavir	0	2	2	May result in reduced atazanavir plasma concentrations.
cefpodoxime proxetil	1	3	2	May result in decreased cefpodoxime effectiveness.
dicumarol	2	3	2	May result in increased or decreased anticoagulant effectiveness.
enoxacin	2	3	2	May result in decreased enoxacin effectiveness.
fosamprenavir	2	3	2	May result in decreased amprenavir serum concentrations (active metabolite of fosamprenavir) and potential reduction of amprenavir efficacy.
gefitinib	0	3	2	May result in reduced plasma concentrations of gefitinib.
glipizide	2	3	2	May result in hypoglycemia.
itraconazole	2	3	2	May result in loss of itraconazole efficacy.
risperidone	0	3	2	May result in increased risperidone bioavailability.

tolazoline	1	2	2	May result in decreased tolazoline effectiveness.
triazolam	0	3	2	May result in increased triazolam absorption and serum concentrations, increasing the risk of triazolam toxicity (excessive sedation, confusion).
warfarin	2	3	2	May result in increased risk of bleeding.
RISEDRONATE				
food	1	3	2	May result in loss of risedronate efficacy.
RISPERIDONE				
Antiarrhythmic Agents, Class IA (*ajmaline, disopyramide, hydroquinidine, moricizine, pirmenol, prajmaline, procainamide, quinidine, recainam*)	0	2	2	May result in increased risk of cardiotoxicity (QT prolongation, torsades de pointes, cardiac arrest).
bupropion	2	3	2	May result in increased plasma levels of risperidone.
carbamazepine	2	3	2	May result in increased risperidone clearance.
cimetidine	0	3	2	May result in increased risperidone bioavailability.
fluoxetine	0	3	2	May result in increased risk of risperidone adverse effects such as serotonin syndrome (hypertension, hyperthermia, myoclonus, mental status changes), extrapyramidal effects, and cardiotoxicity (QT prolongation, torsades de pointes, cardiac arrest) due to increased plasma risperidone levels.

ONSET: 0 - NOT SPECIFIED 1 - RAPID 2 - DELAYED   SEVERITY: 1 - CONTRAINDICATED 2 - MAJOR 3 - MODERATE

itraconazole	2	3	1	May result in increased risperidone concentrations.
lamotrigine	2	3	2	May result in increased risperidone plasma concentrations and risk of adverse effects.
levorphanol	2	3	2	May result in precipitation of opioid withdrawal symptoms in opioid-dependent patients.
linezolid	0	2	2	May result in increased risk of serotonin syndrome (hyperthermia, hyperreflexia, myoclonus, mental status changes).
lithium	2	2	2	May result in weakness, dyskinesias, increased extrapyramidal symptoms, encephalopathy, and brain damage.
methadone	2	3	2	May result in precipitation of opioid withdrawal symptoms in opioid-dependent patients.
paroxetine	2	3	2	May result in increased risk of risperidone adverse effects such as serotonin syndrome (hypertension, hyperthermia, myoclonus, mental status changes), extrapyramidal effects, and cardiotoxicity (QT prolongation, torsades de pointes, cardiac arrest) due to increased plasma risperidone levels.
phenobarbital	2	3	2	May result in decreased plasma concentrations of risperidone and the active metabolite 9-hydroxyrisperidone.
phenytoin	2	3	2	May result in decreased plasma concentrations of risperidone and the active metabolite 9-hydroxyrisperidone.

quetiapine	0	2	2	May result in increased risk of cardiotoxicity (QT prolongation, torsades de pointes, cardiac arrest).
ranitidine	0	3	2	May result in increased risperidone bioavailability.
rifampin	2	3	2	May result in decreased plasma concentrations of risperidone and the active metabolite 9-hydroxyrisperidone.
ritonavir	1	3	2	May result in increased risperidone serum concentrations and potential toxicity (hypotension, sedation, extrapyramidal effects, arrhythmias).
simvastatin	2	2	2	May result in increased simvastatin serum concentrations with an increased risk of myopathy or rhabdomyolysis.
topiramate	0	3	1	May result in decreased risperidone exposure.
ROPINIROLE				
ciprofloxacin	2	3	1	May result in increased risk of ropinirole adverse effects (nausea, somnolence, dizziness).
kava	1	3	2	May result in decreased effectiveness of ropinirole.
tobacco	0	3	2	May result in decreased ropinirole plasma concentrations and efficacy.
ROSIGLITAZONE				
bitter melon	1	3	2	May result in increased risk of hypoglycemia.
fenugreek	1	3	2	May result in increased risk of hypoglycemia.

ONSET: 0 - NOT SPECIFIED 1 - RAPID 2 - DELAYED   SEVERITY: 1 - CONTRAINDICATED 2 - MAJOR 3 - MODERATE

gemfibrozil	1	3	2	May result in increased plasma concentrations of rosiglitazone.
glucomannan	1	3	2	May result in increased risk of hypoglycemia.
guar gum	1	3	2	May result in increased risk of hypoglycemia.
psyllium	1	3	2	May result in increased risk of hypoglycemia.
rifampin	1	3	1	May result in decreased rosiglitazone bioavailability and effectiveness.
St. John's wort	1	3	2	May result in hypoglycemia.
trimethoprim	1	3	1	May result in increased rosiglitazone serum concentrations and risk of hypoglycemia and toxicity (fluid retention, congestive cardiac failure, CNS depression, seizures, diaphoresis, tachypnea, tachycardia, hypothermia).

ROSUVASTATIN

Contraceptives, Combination (*desogestrel, ethinyl estradiol, ethynodiol, etonogestrel, levonorgestrel, mestranol, norelgestromin, norethindrone, norgestimate, norgestrel*)	0	3	2	May result in increased exposure to ethinyl estradiol and norgestrel.
cyclosporine	0	2	2	May result in increased plasma rosuvastatin concentrations and risk of myopathy.
fluconazole	2	3	2	May result in increased rosuvastatin exposure and an increased risk of myopathy or rhabdomyolysis.

itraconazole	2	3	2	May result in increased rosuvastatin exposure and an increased risk of myopathy or rhabdomyolysis.
lopinavir	2	3	1	May result in increased rosuvastatin exposure and maximum concentration.
niacin	2	2	2	May result in increased risk of myopathy or rhabdomyolysis.
oat bran	2	3	2	May result in reduced effectiveness of HMG CoA reductase inhibitors.
pectin	2	3	2	May result in reduced effectiveness of HMG CoA reductase inhibitors.
St. John's wort	2	3	2	May result in reduced effectiveness of rosuvastatin.
warfarin	2	3	2	May result in increased INR and increased risk of bleeding.
SALMETEROL				
erythromycin	2	3	1	May result in increased salmeterol maximum plasma concentration and adverse events.
MAOIs (*clorgyline, iproniazide, isocarboxazid, moclobemide, nialamide, pargyline, phenelzine, procarbazine, selegiline, toloxatone, tranylcypromine*)	2	2	2	May result in increased risk of tachycardia, agitation, or hypomania.

ONSET: 0 = NOT SPECIFIED 1 = RAPID 2 = DELAYED   SEVERITY: 1 = CONTRAINDICATED 2 = MAJOR 3 = MODERATE
EVIDENCE: 1 = EXCELLENT 2 = GOOD

INTERACTING DRUG	ONSET	SEVERITY	EVIDENCE	WARNING
SERTRALINE				
alprazolam	1	3	2	May result in increased risk of psychomotor impairment and sedation.
amitriptyline	2	2	2	May result in elevated amitriptyline serum levels or possible serotonin syndrome (hypertension, hyperthermia, myoclonus, mental status changes).
amoxapine	2	2	2	May result in modest elevation in amoxapine serum levels or possible serotonin syndrome (hypertension, hyperthermia, myoclonus, mental status changes).
Anticoagulants (abciximab, acenocoumarol, ancrod, anisindione, antithrombin III human, bivalirudin, cilostazol, clopidogrel, danaparoid, defibrotide, dermatan sulfate, dicumarol, eptifibatide, fondaparinux, lamifiban, pentosan polysulfate sodium, phenindione, phenprocoumon, sibrafiban, warfarin, xemilofiban)	0	2	2	May result in increased risk of bleeding.
Antiplatelet Agents (abciximab, anagrelide, aspirin, cilostazol, clopidogrel, dipyridamole, epoprostenol, eptifibatide, iloprost, lamifiban, lexipafant, sulfinpyrazone, sulodexide, ticlopidine, tirofiban, xemilofiban)	0	2	2	May result in increased risk of bleeding.

astemizole	1	2	2	May result in cardiotoxicity (QT interval prolongation, torsades de pointes, cardiac arrest).
bupropion	2	3	2	May result in increased plasma levels of sertraline.
carbamazepine	2	3	2	May result in increased risk of carbamazepine toxicity (ataxia, nystagmus, diplopia, headache, vomiting, apnea, seizures, coma).
cimetidine	1	3	2	May result in elevated sertraline serum concentrations and increased risk of adverse side effects.
clomipramine	2	2	2	May result in modest elevations of clomipramine serum levels or possible serotonin syndrome (hypertension, hyperthermia, myoclonus, mental status changes).
clorgyline	1	1	2	May result in CNS toxicity or serotonin syndrome (hypertension, hyperthermia, myoclonus, mental status changes).
clozapine	2	3	2	May result in increased risk of clozapine toxicity (sedation, seizures, hypotension).
darunavir	0	3	1	May result in decreased sertraline exposure and plasma concentrations.
desipramine	2	2	2	May result in modest elevation of desipramine serum levels or possible serotonin syndrome (hypertension, hyperthermia, myoclonus, mental status changes).

ONSET: 0 - NOT SPECIFIED, 1 - RAPID, 2 - DELAYED   SEVERITY: 1 - CONTRAINDICATED, 2 - MAJOR, 3 - MODERATE

dothiepin	2	2	2	May result in modest elevations in dothiepin serum levels or possible serotonin syndrome (hypertension, hyperthermia, myoclonus, mental status changes).
doxepin	2	2	2	May result in modest elevations in doxepin serum levels or possible serotonin syndrome (hypertension, hyperthermia, myoclonus, mental status changes).
eletriptan	2	2	2	May result in increased risk of serotonin syndrome.
erythromycin	2	2	2	May result in increased risk of serotonin syndrome (hypertension, hyperthermia, myoclonus, mental status changes).
flecainide	1	2	2	May result in increased risk of flecainide toxicity (cardiac arrhythmia).
fluphenazine	2	3	2	May result in increased risk of developing acute parkinsonism.
fosphenytoin	2	3	2	May result in increased risk of phenytoin toxicity (ataxia, hyperreflexia, nystagmus, tremor).
frovatriptan	2	2	2	May result in increased risk of serotonin syndrome.
ginkgo	2	3	2	May result in increased risk of serotonin syndrome (hypertension, hyperthermia, myoclonus, mental status changes).
grapefruit juice	2	3	2	May result in elevated sertraline serum concentrations and an increased risk of adverse side effects.

imipramine	2	2	2	May result in modest elevations in imipramine serum levels or possible serotonin syndrome (hypertension, hyperthermia, myoclonus, mental status changes).
iproniazid	1	1	2	May result in CNS toxicity or serotonin syndrome (hypertension, hyperthermia, myoclonus, mental status changes).
isocarboxazid	1	1	2	May result in CNS toxicity or serotonin syndrome (hypertension, hyperthermia, myoclonus, mental status changes).
lamotrigine	2	3	2	May result in increased risk of lamotrigine toxicity (fatigue, sedation, confusion, decreased cognition).
linezolid	1	2	2	May result in CNS toxicity or serotonin syndrome (hypertension, hyperthermia, myoclonus, mental status changes).
lithium	2	3	1	May result in possible increased lithium concentrations and/or an increased risk of SSRI-related serotonin syndrome (hypertension, hyperthermia, myoclonus, mental status changes).
lofepramine	2	2	2	May result in modest elevations in lofepramine serum levels or possible serotonin syndrome (hypertension, hyperthermia, myoclonus, mental status changes).

Drug				Effect
metoclopramide	2	3	2	May result in increased risk of developing extrapyramidal symptoms.
moclobemide	1	1	2	May result in CNS toxicity or serotonin syndrome (hypertension, hyperthermia, myoclonus, mental status changes).
naratriptan	2	2	2	May result in increased risk of serotonin syndrome.
nialamide	1	1	2	May result in CNS toxicity or serotonin syndrome (hypertension, hyperthermia, myoclonus, mental status changes).
nortriptyline	2	2	2	May result in elevated nortriptyline serum levels or possible serotonin syndrome (hypertension, hyperthermia, myoclonus, mental status changes).
NSAIDs (aceclofenac, acemetacin, alclofenac, apazone, benoxaprofen, bromfenac, bufexamac, carprofen, celecoxib, clometacin, clonixin, dexketoprofen, diclofenac, diflunisal, dipyrone, dofetilide, droxicam, etodolac, etofenamate, felbinac, fenbufen, fenoprofen, fentiazac, floctafenine, flufenamic acid, flurbiprofen, ibuprofen, indomethacin, indoprofen, isoxicam, ketoprofen, ketorolac, lornoxicam, meclofenamate, mefanamic acid,	0	3	2	May result in increased risk of bleeding.

meloxicam, nabumetone, naproxen, niflumic acid, nimesulide, oxaprozin, oxyphenbutazone, phenylbutazone, pirazolac, piroxicam, pirprofen, propyphenazon, proquazone, rofecoxib, sulindac, suprofen, tenidap, tenoxicam, tiaprofenic acid, ticrynafen, tolmetin, zomepirac)				
oxycodone	2	2	2	May result in increased risk of serotonin syndrome (tachycardia, hyperthermia, myoclonus, mental status changes).
pargyline	1	1	2	May result in CNS toxicity or serotonin syndrome (hypertension, hyperthermia, myoclonus, mental status changes).
phenelzine	1	1	2	May result in CNS toxicity or serotonin syndrome (hypertension, hyperthermia, myoclonus, mental status changes).
phenytoin	2	3	2	May result in increased risk of phenytoin toxicity (ataxia, hyperreflexia, nystagmus, tremor).
pimozide	0	1	2	May result in increased plasma pimozide levels.
procarbazine	1	1	2	May result in CNS toxicity or serotonin syndrome (hypertension, hyperthermia, myoclonus, mental status changes).

ONSET: 0 = NOT SPECIFIED 1 = RAPID 2 = DELAYED   SEVERITY: 1 = CONTRAINDICATED 2 = MAJOR 3 = MODERATE

propafenone	2	3	2	May result in increased risk of propafenone toxicity (cardiac arrhythmias).
propranolol	2	3	2	May result in increased risk of chest pain.
protriptyline	2	2	2	May result in modest elevations in protriptyline serum levels or possible serotonin syndrome (hypertension, hyperthermia, myoclonus, mental status changes).
rasagiline	0	2	2	May result in CNS toxicity or serotonin syndrome (hypertension, hyperthermia, myoclonus, mental status changes).
rifampin	2	3	2	May result in loss of sertraline efficacy.
rizatriptan	2	2	2	May result in increased risk of serotonin syndrome.
selegiline	1	1	2	May result in CNS toxicity or serotonin syndrome (hypertension, hyperthermia, myoclonus, mental status changes).
sibutramine	1	2	2	May result in increased risk of serotonin syndrome (hypertension, hyperthermia, myoclonus, mental status changes).
St. John's wort	1	2	2	May result in increased risk of serotonin syndrome (hypertension, hyperthermia, myoclonus, mental status changes).
terfenadine	1	2	2	May result in cardiotoxicity (QT prolongation, torsades de pointes, cardiac arrest).

toloxatone	1	1	2	May result in CNS toxicity or serotonin syndrome (hypertension, hyperthermia, myoclonus, mental status changes).
tranylcypromine	1	1	2	May result in CNS toxicity or serotonin syndrome (hypertension, hyperthermia, myoclonus, mental status changes).
trimipramine	2	2	2	May result in modest elevations in trimipramine serum levels or possible serotonin syndrome (hypertension, hyperthermia, myoclonus, mental status changes).
zolmitriptan	2	2	2	May result in increased risk of serotonin syndrome.
zolpidem	2	3	2	May result in increased risk of hallucinations.
SILDENAFIL				
α-1 Blockers (*alfuzosin, bunazosin, doxazosin, moxisylate, phenoxybenzamine, phentolamine, prazosin, tamsulosin, terazosin, trimazosin, urapidil*)	1	3	2	May result in potentiation of hypotensive effects.
amprenavir	1	3	2	May result in increased risk of sildenafil adverse effects (hypotension, visual changes, priapism).
darunavir	0	3	1	May result in increased sildenafil levels.

ONSET: 0 - NOT SPECIFIED, 1 - RAPID, 2 - DELAYED   SEVERITY: 1 - CONTRAINDICATED, 2 - MAJOR, 3 - MODERATE

delavirdine	1	3	2	May result in increased risk of sildenafil adverse effects (hypotension, visual changes, priapism).
dihydrocodeine	0	2	2	May result in increased risk of priapism.
erythromycin	1	3	2	May result in increased risk of sildenafil adverse effects (hypotension, visual changes, priapism).
fosamprenavir	1	3	2	May result in increased risk of sildenafil adverse effects (hypotension, visual changes, priapism).
grapefruit juice	0	3	2	May result in increased sildenafil bioavailability and delayed sildenafil absorption.
indinavir	1	3	2	May result in increased risk of sildenafil adverse effects (hypotension, visual changes, priapism).
itraconazole	2	3	2	May result in increased risk of prolonged sildenafil adverse effects (headache, flushing, priapism).
ketoconazole	2	3	2	May result in increased risk of prolonged sildenafil adverse effects (headache, flushing, priapism).
nelfinavir	1	3	2	May result in increased risk of sildenafil adverse effects (hypotension, visual changes, priapism).
Organic Nitrates (*erythrityl tetranitrate, isosorbide dinitrate, isosorbide mononitrate, nitroglycerin, pentaerythritol tetranitrate*)	1	1	1	May result in potentiation of hypotensive effects.

rifapentine	2	3	2	May result in decreased sildenafil efficacy.
ritonavir	1	2	1	May result in increased risk of sildenafil adverse effects (hypotension, visual changes, priapism).
saquinavir	1	3	1	May result in increased risk of sildenafil adverse effects (hypotension, visual changes, priapism).
SIMVASTATIN				
amiodarone	2	2	1	May result in increased risk of myopathy or rhabdomyolysis.
amprenavir	2	2	2	May result in increased risk of myopathy or rhabdomyolysis.
bosentan	1	3	2	May result in reduced plasma concentrations and reduced efficacy of simvastatin.
carbamazepine	2	3	2	May result in reduced simvastatin exposure.
clarithromycin	2	2	2	May result in increased risk of myopathy or rhabdomyolysis.
conivaptan	0	3	2	May result in increased simvastatin exposure.
cyclosporine	2	2	1	May result in increased risk of myopathy or rhabdomyolysis.

dalfopristin	2	2	2	May result in increased risk of myopathy or rhabdomyolysis.
danazol	2	2	2	May result in increased risk of myopathy or rhabdomyolysis.
digoxin	2	3	2	May result in increased risk of digoxin toxicity (nausea, vomiting, arrhythmias).
diltiazem	1	3	1	May result in increased serum concentration of simvastatin.
efavirenz	2	3	1	May result in decreased simvastatin plasma concentration.
erythromycin	2	2	2	May result in increased risk of myopathy or rhabdomyolysis.
fluconazole	2	2	2	May result in increased risk of myopathy or rhabdomyolysis.
fosphenytoin	2	3	2	May result in loss of simvastatin efficacy.
fusidic acid	2	2	2	May result in increased risk of myopathy or rhabdomyolysis.
gemfibrozil	2	2	2	May result in increased risk of myopathy or rhabdomyolysis.

grapefruit juice	1	2	1	May result in increased bioavailability of simvastatin resulting in increased risk of myopathy or rhabdomyolysis.
imatinib	2	3	2	May result in increased plasma concentrations of simvastatin.
indinavir	2	2	2	May result in increased risk of myopathy or rhabdomyolysis.
itraconazole	2	1	2	May result in increased risk of myopathy or rhabdomyolysis.
ketoconazole	2	2	2	May result in increased risk of myopathy or rhabdomyolysis.
mibefradil	2	1	2	May result in increased risk of myopathy and/or rhabdomyolysis.
nefazodone	2	2	2	May result in increased risk of myopathy or rhabdomyolysis.
nelfinavir	2	2	2	May result in increased risk of myopathy or rhabdomyolysis.
niacin	2	2	2	May result in increased risk of myopathy or rhabdomyolysis.

ONSET: 0 - NOT SPECIFIED, 1 - RAPID, 2 - DELAYED   SEVERITY: 1 - CONTRAINDICATED, 2 - MAJOR, 3 - MODERATE

oat bran	2	3	2	May result in reduced effectiveness of HMG CoA reductase inhibitors.
oxcarbazepine	2	3	2	May result in reduced simvastatin exposure.
pectin	2	3	2	May result in reduced effectiveness of HMG CoA reductase inhibitors.
phenytoin	2	3	2	May result in loss of simvastatin efficacy.
quinupristin	2	2	2	May result in increased risk of myopathy or rhabdomyolysis.
ranolazine	0	3	2	May result in increased simvastatin plasma concentrations.
rifampin	2	3	2	May result in decreased simvastatin effectiveness.
risperidone	2	2	2	May result in increased simvastatin serum concentrations with an increased risk of myopathy or rhabdomyolysis.
ritonavir	2	2	2	May result in increased risk of myopathy or rhabdomyolysis.
saquinavir	2	2	2	May result in increased risk of myopathy or rhabdomyolysis.
St. John's wort	2	3	2	May result in reduced effectiveness of simvastatin.
telithromycin	2	2	2	May result in increased simvastatin plasma levels.
verapamil	2	2	2	May result in increased risk of myopathy or rhabdomyolysis.

voriconazole	0	3	2	May result in increased plasma concentrations of simvastatin.
warfarin	2	3	1	May result in increased risk of bleeding and an increased risk of rhabdomyolysis.

SITAGLIPTIN

none reported

SPIRONOLACTONE

ACE Inhibitors (*alacepril, benazepril, captopril, cilazapril, delapril, enalapril maleate, enalaprilat, fosinopril, imidapril, lisinopril, moexipril, pentopril, perindopril, quinapril, ramipril, spirapril, temocapril, trandolapril, zofenopril*)	2	2	2	May result in hyperkalemia.
arginine	1	2	2	May result in potentially fatal hyperkalemia.
digitoxin	2	3	2	May result in increased or decreased digitoxin elimination.
digoxin	2	2	2	May result in digoxin toxicity (nausea, vomiting, cardiac arrhythmias).
gossypol	2	3	2	May result in increased risk of hypokalemia.
licorice	2	3	2	May result in increased risk of hypokalemia and/or reduced effectiveness of the diuretic.

ONSET: 0 - NOT SPECIFIED 1 - RAPID 2 - DELAYED   SEVERITY: 1 - CONTRAINDICATED 2 - MAJOR 3 - MODERATE

NSAIDs (*aceclofenac, acemetacin, alclofenac, apazone, aspirin, benoxaprofen, bromfenac, bufexamac, carprofen, celecoxib, clometacin, clonixin, dexketoprofen, diclofenac, diflunisal, dipyrone, dofetilide, droxicam, etodolac, etofenamate, felbinac, fenbufen, fenoprofen, fentiazac, floctafe nine, flufenamic acid, flurbiprofen, ibuprofen, indomethacin, indoprofen, isoxicam, ketoprofen, ketorolac, lornoxicam, meclofenamate, mefanamic acid, meloxicam, nabumetone, naproxen, niflumic acid, nimesulide, oxaprozin, oxyphenbutazone, phenylbutazone, pirazolac, piroxicam, pirprofen, propyphenazon, proquazone, rofecoxib, sulindac, suprofen, tenidap, tenoxicam, tiaprofenic acid, ticrynafen, tolmetin, zomepirac)*	2	3	2	May result in reduced diuretic effectiveness, hyperkalemia, or possible nephrotoxicity.
sotalol	0	2	2	May result in increased risk of cardiotoxicity (QT prolongation, torsades de pointes, cardiac arrest).

SULFAMETHOXAZOLE

acetohexamide	2	3	2	May result in enhanced hypoglycemic effects.

	Onset	Severity	Documentation	
anisindione	2	3	2	May result in increased risk of bleeding.
Antiarrhythmic Agents, Class IA (*ajmaline, disopyramide, hydroquinidine, moricizine, pirmenol, prajmaline, procainamide, quinidine, recainam*)	0	2	2	May result in increased risk of cardiotoxicity (QT prolongation, torsades de pointes, cardiac arrest).
chlorpropamide	2	3	2	May result in enhanced hypoglycemic effects.
dofetilide	0	1	2	May result in increased risk of cardiotoxicity (QT prolongation, torsades de pointes, cardiac arrest).
ethanol	1	2	2	May result in disulfiram-like reaction (flushing, sweating, palpitations, drowsiness).
glipizide	2	3	2	May result in enhanced hypoglycemic effects.
glyburide	2	3	2	May result in enhanced hypoglycemic effects.
methotrexate	2	2	1	May result in increased risk of methotrexate toxicity (myelotoxicity, pancytopenia, megaloblastic anemia).
pyrimethamine	2	2	2	May result in increased risk of megaloblastic anemia and pancytopenia.
rifabutin	2	3	2	May result in increased sulfamethoxazole hydroxylamine exposure.

TCAs (*amitriptyline, amitriptylinoxide, amoxapine, clomipramine, desipramine, dibenzepin, dothiepin, doxepin, imipramine, lofepramine, melitracen, nortriptyline, opipramol, protriptyline, tianeptine, trimipramine*)	0	2	2	May result in increased risk of cardiotoxicity (QT prolongation, torsades de pointes, cardiac arrest).
tolazamide	2	3	2	May result in enhanced hypoglycemic effects.
tolbutamide	2	3	2	May result in enhanced hypoglycemic effects.
warfarin	2	2	2	May result in increased risk of bleeding.
SUMATRIPTAN				
citalopram	2	2	1	May result in increased risk of serotonin syndrome.
ergonovine	1	1	2	May result in prolonged vasospastic reactions.
ergotamine	1	1	2	May result in prolonged vasospastic reactions.
escitalopram	2	2	2	May result in increased risk of serotonin syndrome.
fluoxetine	2	2	2	May result in increased risk of serotonin syndrome.
fluvoxamine	2	2	2	May result in increased risk of serotonin syndrome.
frovatriptan	1	1	2	May result in prolonged vasospastic reactions.
MAOIs (*clorgyline, iproniazide, isocarboxazid, moclobemide, nialamide, pargyline, phenelzine, procarbazine, selegiline, toloxatone, tranylcypromine*)	1	1	2	May result in increased risk of serotonin syndrome (hypertension, hyperthermia, myoclonus, mental status changes).

	1	1	2	May result in prolonged vasospastic reactions.
methysergide	1	1	2	May result in prolonged vasospastic reactions.
naratriptan	1	1	2	May result in increased risk of serotonin syndrome.
paroxetine	2	2	2	May result in increased risk of serotonin syndrome.
sibutramine	1	2	2	May result in increased risk of serotonin syndrome (hypertension, hypothermia, myoclonus, mental status changes).
zolmitriptan	1	1	2	May result in prolonged vasospastic reactions.
TADALAFIL				
alfuzosin	1	3	2	May result in potentiation of hypotensive effects.
amprenavir	1	3	2	May result in increased tadalafil bioavailability and risk of adverse effects.
doxazosin	1	2	2	May result in potentiation of hypotensive effects.
ethanol	1	3	2	May result in increased risk of hypotension and orthostatic signs and symptoms.
ketoconazole	1	3	2	May result in increased tadalafil bioavailability.
ritonavir	1	3	2	May result in increased tadalafil bioavailability.
tamsulosin	1	3	2	May result in potentiation of hypotensive effects.

TAMSULOSIN

Drug				Effect
β-Blockers (acebutolol, alprenolol, atenolol, betaxolol, bevantolol, bisoprolol, bucindolol, carteolol, carvedilol, celiprolol, dilevalol, esmolol, labetalol, levobunolol, mepindolol, metipranolol, metoprolol, nadolol, nebivolol, oxprenolol, penbutolol, pindolol, propranolol, sotalol, talinolol, tertatolol, timolol)	1	3	2	May result in exaggerated hypotensive response to the first dose of the α-blocker.
cimetidine	1	3	2	May result in increased risk of tamsulosin toxicity (orthostatic hypotension, dizziness, syncope).
sildenafil	1	3	2	May result in potentiation of hypotensive effects.
sotalol	1	3	2	May result in exaggerated hypotensive response to the first dose of the α-blocker.
tadalafil	1	3	2	May result in potentiation of hypotensive effects.
vardenafil	1	2	1	May result in potentiation of hypotensive effects.

TEMAZEPAM

Drug				Effect
Barbiturates (amobarbital, aprobarbital, butabarbital, butalbital, mephobarbital, methohexital, pentobarbital, phenobarbital, primidone, secobarbital, thiopental)	0	2	2	May result in additive respiratory depression.

ethanol	1	3	2	May result in impaired psychomotor functions.
Opioid Analgesics (*alfentanil, anileridine, codeine, fentanyl, hydrocodone, hydromorphone, levorphanol, meperidine, morphine, morphine sulfate liposome, oxycodone, oxymorphone, propoxyphene, remifentanil, sufentanil*)	0	2	2	May result in additive respiratory depression.
rifapentine	2	3	2	May result in reduced diazepam plasma concentrations and effectiveness.
St. John's wort	2	3	2	May result in reduced BZD effectiveness.
theophylline	1	3	2	May result in decreased BZD effectiveness.
TERAZOSIN				
β-Blockers (*acebutolol, alprenolol, atenolol, betaxolol, bevantolol, bisoprolol, bucindolol, carteolol, carvedilol, celiprolol, dilevalol, esmolol, labetalol, levobunolol, mepindolol, metipranolol, metoprolol, nadolol, nebivolol, oxprenolol, penbutolol, pindolol, propranolol, sotalol, talinolol, tertatolol, timolol*)	1	3	2	May result in exaggerated hypotensive response to the first dose of the α-blocker.

ONSET: 0 – NOT SPECIFIED, 1 – RAPID, 2 – DELAYED.   SEVERITY: 1 – CONTRAINDICATED, 2 – MAJOR, 3 – MODERATE.

sildenafil	1	3	2	May result in potentiation of hypotensive effects.
vardenafil	1	2	1	May result in potentiation of hypotensive effects.
TIZANIDINE				
ciprofloxacin	1	1	1	May result in increased tizanidine plasma concentrations resulting in increased hypotensive and sedative effects.
Contraceptives, Combination (*ethinyl estradiol, mestranol*)	1	2	2	May result in increased tizanidine plasma concentrations resulting in increased hypotensive and sedative effects.
fluvoxamine	1	1	1	May result in increased tizanidine bioavailability and an increased risk of tizanidine adverse effects (profound hypotension, bradycardia, excessive drowsiness).
fosphenytoin	2	3	2	May result in increased risk of phenytoin toxicity (ataxia, hyperreflexia, nystagmus, tremor).
lisinopril	1	3	2	May result in potentiation of hypotensive response.
phenytoin	2	3	2	May result in increased risk of phenytoin toxicity (ataxia, hyperreflexia, nystagmus, tremor).
TOLTERODINE				
clarithromycin	1	3	2	May result in enhanced tolterodine bioavailability in individuals with deficient cytochrome P450 2D6 activity.
cyclosporine	1	3	2	May result in enhanced tolterodine bioavailability in individuals with deficient cytochrome P450 2D6 activity.

erythromycin	1	3	2	May result in enhanced tolterodine bioavailability in individuals with deficient cytochrome P450 2D6 activity.
itraconazole	1	3	2	May result in enhanced tolterodine bioavailability in individuals with deficient cytochrome P450 2D6 activity.
ketoconazole	1	3	2	May result in enhanced tolterodine bioavailability in individuals with deficient cytochrome P450 2D6 activity.
miconazole	1	3	2	May result in enhanced tolterodine bioavailability in individuals with deficient cytochrome P450 2D6 activity.
vinblastine	1	3	2	May result in enhanced tolterodine bioavailability in individuals with deficient cytochrome P450 2D6 activity.
warfarin	2	3	2	May result in increased risk of bleeding.
TOPIRAMATE				
carbamazepine	2	3	2	May result in decreased topiramate concentrations.
Contraceptives, Combination (*desogestrel, ethinyl estradiol, ethynodiol, etonogestrel, levonorgestrel, mestranol, norelgestromin, norethindrone, norgestimate, norgestrel*)	2	3	2	May result in reduced contraceptive efficacy.
fosphenytoin	2	3	2	May result in altered topiramate or phenytoin concentrations.
ginkgo	2	3	2	May result in decreased anticonvulsant effectiveness.
HCTZ	2	3	2	May result in increased topiramate exposure.

ONSET: 0 - NOT SPECIFIED, 1 - RAPID, 2 - DELAYED   SEVERITY: 1 - CONTRAINDICATED, 2 - MAJOR, 3 - MODERATE

metformin	0	3	2	May result in increased metformin and topiramate exposure.
phenobarbital	2	3	2	May result in decreased serum concentrations of topiramate.
phenytoin	2	3	2	May result in altered topiramate or phenytoin concentrations.
pioglitazone	2	3	2	May result in decreased pioglitazone exposure.
risperidone	0	3	1	May result in decreased risperidone exposure.
valproic acid	2	3	2	May result in decreased topiramate or valproic acid concentrations, and increased risk of encephalopathy.
TRAMADOL				
carbamazepine	0	2	2	May result in decreased tramadol efficacy and increased seizure risk.
digoxin	2	3	2	May result in increased risk of digoxin toxicity (nausea, vomiting, cardiac arrhythmias).
fluoxetine	1	2	2	May result in increased risk of seizures and serotonin syndrome (hypertension, hyperthermia, myoclonus, mental status changes); increased concentrations of tramadol and decreased concentrations of tramadol active metabolite, M1.

linezolid	0	2	2	May result in increased risk of serotonin syndrome (hyperthermia, hyperreflexia, myoclonus, mental status changes).
mirtazapine	2	2	2	May result in increased risk of serotonin syndrome (tachycardia, hyperthermia, myoclonus, mental status changes).
quinidine	0	3	2	May result in increased concentrations of tramadol and decreased concentrations of tramadol active metabolite, M1.
warfarin	2	3	2	May result in increased prothrombin time and an increased risk of bleeding.
TRAZODONE				
amiodarone	2	2	2	May result in increased risk of QT interval prolongation and torsade de pointes.
atazanavir	0	3	2	May result in increased trazodone plasma levels and increased risk of trazodone side effects (nausea, dizziness, hypotension).
carbamazepine	2	3	2	May result in decreased trazodone plasma concentrations.
chlorpromazine	2	3	2	May result in hypotension.

digoxin	2	3	2	May result in increased digoxin serum concentrations and an increased risk of digoxin toxicity (nausea, vomiting, arrhythmias).
fluoxetine	2	2	2	May result in trazodone toxicity (sedation, dry mouth, urinary retention) or serotonin syndrome (hypertension, hyperthermia, myoclonus, mental status changes).
foxglove	2	3	2	May result in increased risk of digitalis toxicity.
ginkgo	1	2	2	May result in excessive sedation and potential coma.
indinavir	0	3	2	May result in increased trazodone plasma levels.
itraconazole	0	3	2	May result in increased trazodone serum concentrations.
ketoconazole	0	3	2	May result in increased trazodone plasma levels.
nefazodone	0	3	2	May result in increased trazodone serum concentrations.
paroxetine	1	2	2	May result in serotonin syndrome (hypertension, hyperthermia, myoclonus, mental status changes).
phenytoin	0	3	2	May result in increased phenytoin serum concentrations and an increased risk of phenytoin toxicity (ataxia, hyperreflexia, nystagmus, tremor).

ritonavir	0	3	2	May result in increased trazodone plasma levels and increased risk of trazodone side effects.
St. John's wort	2	2	2	May result in increased risk of serotonin syndrome (hypertension, hyerthermia, myoclonus, mental status changes).
thioridazine	2	3	2	May result in hypotension.
tipranavir	0	3	2	May result in increased plasma concentrations of trazodone and increased risk of trazodone adverse effects (nausea, dizziness, hypotension, syncope).
trifluoperazine	2	3	2	May result in hypotension.
TRIAMCINOLONE				
alcuronium	2	3	2	May result in decreased alcuronium effectiveness; prolonged muscle weakness and myopathy.
aspirin	2	3	2	May result in increased risk of gastrointestinal ulceration and subtherapeutic aspirin serum concentrations.
atracurium	2	3	2	May result in decreased atracurium effectiveness; prolonged muscle weakness and myopathy.

ONSET: 0 = NOT SPECIFIED 1 = RAPID 2 = DELAYED   SEVERITY: 1 = CONTRAINDICATED 2 = MAJOR 3 = MODERATE
EVIDENCE: 1 = EXCELLENT 2 = GOOD

305/TRIAMCINOLONE

INTERACTING DRUG	ONSET	SEVERITY	EVIDENCE	WARNING
FLQs (alatrofloxacin, balofloxacin, cinoxacin, ciprofloxacin, clinafloxacin, enoxacin, fleroxacin, flumequine, gemifloxacin, grepafloxacin, levofloxacin, lomefloxacin, moxifloxacin, norfloxacin, ofloxacin, pefloxacin, prulifloxacin, rosoxacin, rufloxacin, sparfloxacin, temafloxacin, tosufloxacin, trovafloxacin)	2	3	1	May result in increased risk for tendon rupture.
gallamine	2	3	2	May result in decreased gallamine effectiveness; prolonged muscle weakness and myopathy.
hexafluorenium	2	3	2	May result in decreased hexafluorenium bromide effectiveness; prolonged muscle weakness and myopathy.
itraconazole	2	3	2	May result in increased corticosteroid plasma concentrations and an increased risk of corticosteroid side effects (myopathy, glucose intolerance, Cushing's syndrome).
licorice	2	3	2	May result in increased risk of corticosteroid adverse effects.
metocurine	2	3	2	May result in decreased metocurine effectiveness; prolonged muscle weakness and myopathy.
phenytoin	2	3	2	May result in decreased triamcinolone effectiveness.
primidone	2	3	2	May result in decreased triamcinolone effectiveness.

quetiapine	0	2	2	May result in decreased serum quetiapine concentrations.
rotavirus vaccine, live	2	1	1	May result in increased risk of infection by the live vaccine.
saiboku-to	2	3	2	May result in enhanced and prolonged effect of corticosteroids.

TRIAMTERENE

ACE Inhibitors (*alacepril, benazepril, captopril, cilazapril, delapril, enalapril maleate, enalaprilat, fosinopril, imidapril, lisinopril, moexipril, pentopril, perindopril, quinapril, ramipril, spirapril, temocapril, trandolapril, zofenopril*)	2	3	2	May result in reduced diuretic effectiveness, hyperkalemia, or possible nephrotoxicity.
amantadine	2	3	2	May result in amantadine toxicity (incoordination, agitation, visual hallucinations).
dofetilide	2	2	2	May result in increased risk of cardiotoxicity (QT prolongation, torsades de pointes, cardiac arrest).
gossypol	2	3	2	May result in increased risk of hypokalemia.
licorice	2	3	2	May result in increased risk of hypokalemia and/or reduced effectiveness of the diuretic.
methotrexate	2	2	2	May result in bone marrow suppression.

ONSET: 0 – NOT SPECIFIED 1 – RAPID 2 – DELAYED   SEVERITY: 1 – CONTRAINDICATED 2 – MAJOR 3 – MODERATE

	2	3	2	
NSAIDs (*aceclofenac, acemetacin, alclofenac, apazone, aspirin, benoxaprofen, bromfenac, bufexamac, carprofen, celecoxib, clometacin, clonixin, dexketoprofen, diclofenac, diflunisal, dipyrone, dofetilide, droxicam, etodolac, etofenamate, felbinac, fenbufen, fenoprofen, fentiazac, floctafenine, flufenamic acid, flurbiprofen, ibuprofen, indomethacin, indoprofen, isoxicam, ketoprofen, ketorolac, lornoxicam, meclofenamate, mefanamic acid, meloxicam, nabumetone, naproxen, niflumic acid, nimesulide, oxaprozin, oxyphenbutazone, phenylbutazone, pirazolac, piroxicam, pirprofen, propyphenazon, proquazone, rofecoxib, sulindac, suprofen, tenidap, tenoxicam, tiaprofenic acid, ticrynafen, tolmetin, zomepirac*)*	2	3	2	May result in reduced diuretic effectiveness, hyperkalemia, or possible nephrotoxicity.
potassium-containing food	2	3	2	May result in hyperkalemia.
quinidine measurement	0	3	2	May result in interference with fluorescent measurement of quinidine due to similar fluorescence spectra.

ramipril	2	2	2	May result in hyperkalemia.
sotalol	0	2	2	May result in increased risk of cardiotoxicity (QT prolongation, torsades de pointes, cardiac arrest).
TRIMETHOPRIM				
anisindione	2	3	2	May result in increased risk of bleeding.
Antiarrhythmic Agents, Class IA (*ajmaline, disopyramide, hydroquinidine, moricizine, pirmenol, prajmaline, procainamide, quinidine, recainam*)	0	2	2	May result in increased risk of cardiotoxicity (QT prolongation, torsades de pointes, cardiac arrest).
digoxin	2	3	2	May result in increased risk of digoxin toxicity.
dofetilide	0	1	2	May result in increased risk of cardiotoxicity (QT prolongation, torsades de pointes, cardiac arrest).
enalapril maleate	2	3	2	May result in hyperkalemia.
enalaprilat	2	3	2	May result in hyperkalemia.
ethanol	1	2	2	May result in disulfiram-like reaction (flushing, sweating, palpitations, drowsiness).
fosphenytoin	2	3	2	May result in increased risk of phenytoin toxicity (ataxia, nystagmus, hyperreflexia, lethargy).
gemifloxacin	0	2	2	May result in increased risk of cardiotoxicity (QT prolongation, torsades de pointes, cardiac arrest).

ONSET: 0 - NOT SPECIFIED 1 - RAPID 2 - DELAYED   SEVERITY: 1 - CONTRAINDICATED 2 - MAJOR 3 - MODERATE

methotrexate	2	2	1	May result in increased risk of methotrexate toxicity (myelotoxicity, pancytopenia, megaloblastic anemia).
methotrexate measurement	0	3	2	May result in interference with serum methotrexate assay using the competitive binding protein technique due to assay interference.
phenytoin	2	3	2	May result in increased risk of phenytoin toxicity (ataxia, hyperreflexia, nystagmus, tremors).
pyrimethamine	2	2	2	May result in increased risk of megaloblastic anemia and pancytopenia.
quinapril	2	3	2	May result in hyperkalemia.
repaglinide	0	3	2	May result in increased repaglinide exposure and plasma concentration.
rosiglitazone	1	3	1	May result in increased rosiglitazone serum concentrations and risk of hypoglycemia and toxicity (fluid retention, congestive cardiac failure, CNS depression, seizures, diaphoresis, tachypnea, tachycardia, hypothermia).
TCAs (*amitriptyline, amitriptylinoxide, amoxapine, clomipramine, desipramine, dibenzepin, dothiepin, doxepin, imipramine, lofepramine, melitracen, nortriptyline, opipramol, protriptyline, tianeptine, trimipramine*)	0	2	2	May result in increased risk of cardiotoxicity (QT prolongation, torsades de pointes, cardiac arrest).

tolbutamide	2	3	2	May result in enhanced hypoglycemic effects.
trimipramine	0	2	2	May result in increased risk of cardiotoxicity (QT prolongation, torsades de pointes, cardiac arrest).

VALACYCLOVIR

mycophenolate mofetil	0	3	2	May result in increased risk of neutropenia.
mycophenolic acid	0	3	2	May result in increased risk of neutropenia.

VALPROIC ACID

acyclovir	2	3	2	May result in decreased valproic acid plasma concentrations and potential increased seizure activity.
aspirin	2	3	2	May result in increased free valproic acid concentrations.
betamipron	2	3	2	May result in decreased valproic acid efficacy.
carbamazepine	2	3	2	May result in carbamazepine toxicity (ataxia, nystagmus, diplopia, headache, vomiting, apnea, seizures, coma) and/or decreased valproic acid effectiveness.
cholestyramine	1	3	2	May result in decreased serum valproic acid concentrations.
clomipramine	2	3	2	May result in increased risk of clomipramine toxicity (agitation, confusion, hallucinations, urinary retention, tachycardia, seizures, coma).
erythromycin	2	3	2	May result in valproic acid toxicity (CNS depression, seizures).

ONSET: 0 - NOT SPECIFIED, 1 - RAPID, 2 - DELAYED   SEVERITY: 1 - CONTRAINDICATED, 2 - MAJOR, 3 - MODER

ethosuximide	2	3	2	May result in increased risk of ethosuximide toxicity.
felbamate	2	3	2	May result in increased valproic acid concentrations.
fosphenytoin	2	3	2	May result in altered valproate levels or altered phenytoin levels.
ginkgo	2	3	2	May result in decreased anticonvulsant effectiveness.
lamotrigine	2	2	1	May result in increased elimination half-life of lamotrigine leading to lamotrigine toxicity (fatigue, drowsiness, ataxia) and an increased risk of life-threatening rashes.
lopinavir	2	3	2	May result in decreased valproic acid serum concentrations.
lorazepam	1	3	2	May result in increased lorazepam concentrations.
mefloquine	2	3	2	May result in loss of seizure control.
meropenem	1	3	2	May result in decreased valproic acid plasma concentrations and loss of anticonvulsant effect.
nimodipine	2	3	2	May result in nimodipine toxicity (dizziness, headache, flushing, peripheral edema).
nortriptyline	2	3	2	May result in increased serum nortriptyline levels.
oxcarbazepine	0	3	2	May result in decreased plasma concentration of the active 10-monohydroxy metabolite of oxcarbazepine.
panipenem	2	3	2	May result in decreased valproic acid efficacy.

phenobarbital	2	3	2	May result in phenobarbital toxicity or decreased valproic acid effectiveness.
phenytoin	2	3	2	May result in altered valproate levels or altered phenytoin levels.
primidone	1	2	2	May result in severe CNS depression.
rifampin	2	3	2	May result in reduced valproate levels.
rifapentine	2	3	2	May result in decreased anticonvulsant effectiveness.
ritonavir	2	3	2	May result in decreased valproic acid serum concentrations.
topiramate	2	3	2	May result in decreased topiramate or valproic acid concentrations, and increased risk of encephalopathy.
vorinostat	0	2	2	May result in severe thrombocytopenia and gastrointestinal bleeding.
zidovudine	2	3	2	May result in increased zidovudine plasma concentrations and potential zidovudine toxicity (asthenia, fatigue, nausea, hematologic abnormalities).
VALSARTAN				
lithium	2	2	2	May result in increased risk of lithium toxicity (weakness, tremor, excessive thirst, confusion).

ONSET: 0 = NOT SPECIFIED, 1 = RAPID, 2 = DELAYED   SEVERITY: 1 = CONTRAINDICATED, 2 = MAJOR, 3 = MODERATE

VARENICLINE

none reported

VENLAFAXINE

Anticoagulants (*abciximab, acenocoumarol, ancrod, anisindione, antithrombin III human, bivalirudin, cilostazol, clopidogrel, danaparoid, defibrotide, dermatan sulfate, dicumarol, eptifibatide, fondaparinux, lamifiban, pentosan polysulfate sodium, phenindione, phenprocoumon, sibrafiban, warfarin, xemilofiban*)	0	2	2	May result in an increased risk of bleeding.
Antiplatelet Agents (*abciximab, anagrelide, aspirin, cilostazol, clopidogrel, dipyridamole, epoprostenol, eptifibatide, iloprost, lamifiban, lexipafant, sulfinpyrazone, sulodexide, ticlopidine, tirofiban, xemilofiban*)	0	2	2	May result in an increased risk of bleeding.
clozapine	1	3	2	May result in increased serum concentrations of clozapine and venlafaxine.

ginkgo	2	3	2	May result in increased risk of serotonin syndrome (hypertension, hyperthermia, myoclonus, mental status changes).
haloperidol	1	2	2	May result in increased haloperidol serum concentrations and increased risk of cardiotoxicity (QT prolongation, torsades de pointes, cardiac arrest).
iproniazid	1	1	2	May result in CNS toxicity or serotonin syndrome (hypertension, hyperthermia, myoclonus, mental status changes).
isocarboxazid	1	1	2	May result in CNS toxicity or serotonin syndrome (hypertension, hyperthermia, myoclonus, mental status changes).
metoclopramide	2	3	2	May result in increased risk of developing extrapyramidal symptoms.
moclobemide	1	1	2	May result in CNS toxicity or serotonin syndrome (hypertension, hyperthermia, myoclonus, mental status changes).
naratriptan	2	2	2	May result in increased risk of serotonin syndrome.
nialamide	1	1	2	May result in CNS toxicity or serotonin syndrome (hypertension, hyperthermia, myoclonus, mental status changes).

ONSET: 0 - NOT SPECIFIED 1 - RAPID 2 - DELAYED   SEVERITY: 1 - CONTRAINDICATED 2 - MAJOR 3 - MODERATE

Drug				Effect
NSAIDs (aceclofenac, acemetacin, alclofenac, apazone, aspirin, benoxaprofen, bromfenac, bufexamac, carprofen, celecoxib, clometacin, clonixin, dexketoprofen, diclofenac, diflunisal, dipyrone, dofetilide, droxicam, etodolac, etofenamate, felbinac, fenbufen, fenoprofen, fentiazac, floctafenine, flufenamic acid, flurbiprofen, ibuprofen, indomethacin, indoprofen, isoxicam, ketoprofen, ketorolac, lornoxicam, meclofenamate, mefanamic acid, meloxicam, nabumetone, naproxen, niflumic acid, nimesulide, oxaprozin, oxyphenbutazone, phenylbutazone, pirazolac, piroxicam, pirprofen, propyphenazon, proquazone, rofecoxib, sulindac, suprofen, tenidap, tenoxicam, tiaprofenic acid, ticrynafen, tolmetin, zomepirac)	0	3	2	May result in increased risk of bleeding.
pargyline	1	1	2	May result in CNS toxicity or serotonin syndrome (hypertension, hyperthermia, myoclonus, mental status changes).

phenelzine	1	1	2	May result in CNS toxicity or serotonin syndrome (hypertension, hyperthermia, myoclonus, mental status changes).
procarbazine	1	1	2	May result in CNS toxicity or serotonin syndrome (hypertension, hyperthermia, myoclonus, mental status changes).
rizatriptan	2	2	2	May result in increased risk of serotonin syndrome.
selegiline	1	1	2	May result in CNS toxicity or serotonin syndrome (hypertension, hyperthermia, myoclonus, mental status changes).
sibutramine	1	2	2	May result in increased risk of serotonin syndrome (hypertension, hyperthermia, myoclonus, mental status changes).
St. John's wort	2	3	2	May result in increased risk of serotonin syndrome (hypertension, hyperthermia, myoclonus, mental status changes).
toloxatone	1	1	2	May result in CNS toxicity or serotonin syndrome (hypertension, hyperthermia, myoclonus, mental status changes).
tranylcypromine	1	1	2	May result in CNS toxicity or serotonin syndrome (hypertension, hyperthermia, myoclonus, mental status changes).

ONSET: 0 = NOT SPECIFIED 1 = RAPID 2 = DELAYED   SEVERITY: 1 = CONTRAINDICATED 2 = MAJOR 3 = MODERATE
EVIDENCE: 1 = EXCELLENT 2 = GOOD

INTERACTING DRUG	ONSET	SEVERITY	EVIDENCE	WARNING
trifluoperazine	1	1	2	May result in increased risk of neuroleptic malignant syndrome and increased risk of cardiotoxicity (QT prolongation, torsades de pointes, cardiac arrest).
zolpidem	2	3	2	May result in increased risk of hallucinations.
VERAPAMIL				
amiodarone	1	2	2	May result in bradycardia, atrioventricular block and/or sinus arrest.
aspirin	2	3	2	May result in increased risk of bleeding.
β-Blockers (*acebutolol, alprenolol, atenolol, betaxolol, bevantolol, bisoprolol, bucindolol, carteolol, carvedilol, celiprolol, dilevalol, esmolol, labetalol, levobunolol, mepindolol, metipranolol, metoprolol, nadolol, nebivolol, oxprenolol, penbutolol, pindolol, propranolol, sotalol, talinolol, tertatolol, timolol*)	1	2	2	May result in hypotension, bradycardia.
bupivacaine	1	2	2	May result in increased risk of heart block.
buspirone	1	3	2	May result in increased risk of enhanced buspirone effects.
carbamazepine	2	3	2	May result in increased carbamazepine plasma concentrations and risk of toxicity (ataxia, nystagmus, diplopia, headache, vomiting, apnea, seizures, coma).

clarithromycin	2	3	2	May result in increased verapamil plasma concentrations and increased risk of hypotension and/or bradycardia.
cyclosporine	2	3	2	May result in increased risk of cyclosporine toxicity (renal dysfunction, cholestasis, paresthesias).
dalfopristin	2	3	2	May result in increased risk of verapamil toxicity (dizziness, headache, flushing, peripheral edema).
dantrolene	1	2	2	May result in hyperkalemia and cardiac depression.
digitoxin	2	3	2	May result in increased serum digitoxin concentrations or toxicity (nausea, vomiting, cardiac arrhythmias).
digoxin	2	2	1	May result in increased serum digoxin concentrations and toxicity (nausea, vomiting, arrhythmias).
dofetilide	2	1	2	May result in increased risk of cardiotoxicity (QT prolongation, torsades de pointes, cardiac arrest).
dutasteride	0	3	2	May result in increased dutasteride plasma concentrations.
eplerenone	0	2	2	May result in increased eplerenone plasma concentrations and increased risk of eplerenone side effects.
erythromycin	0	2	2	May result in increased risk of cardiotoxicity (QT prolongation, torsades de pointes, bradycardia, hypotension, cardiac arrest).
ethanol	1	3	1	May result in enhanced ethanol intoxication (impaired psychomotor functioning).

ONSET: 0 - NOT SPECIFIED 1 - RAPID 2 - DELAYED   SEVERITY: 1 - CONTRAINDICATED 2 - MAJOR 3 - MODERATE

fentanyl	1	2	2	May result in severe hypotension.
flecainide	1	3	2	May result in excessive negative inotropic effects and prolongation of atrioventricular conduction.
fosphenytoin	2	3	2	May result in decreased verapamil effectiveness.
grapefruit juice	1	3	1	May result in increased risk of verapamil adverse effects (flushing, edema, hypotension, myocardial ischemia).
indinavir	0	3	2	May result in increased plasma concentrations of CCB.
itraconazole	2	3	2	May result in increased verapamil serum concentrations and toxicity (dizziness, hypotension, flushing, headache, peripheral edema).
lithium	2	3	2	May result in loss of mania control, neurotoxicity, bradycardia.
mepivacaine	1	2	2	May result in increased risk of heart block.
midazolam	1	3	2	May result in increased/prolonged sedation.
nevirapine	0	3	2	May result in decreased plasma concentrations of verapamil.
oxcarbazepine	2	3	1	May result in decreased plasma levels of the active 10-monohydroxy metabolite of oxcarbazepine and potential loss of oxcarbazepine efficacy.
pancuronium	1	3	2	May result in enhanced neuromuscular blockade.
phenobarbital	2	3	2	May result in decreased verapamil effectiveness.

phenytoin	2	3	2	May result in decreased verapamil effectiveness.
quinidine	1	3	2	May result in hypotension, counteraction by verapamil of quinidine's effect on AV conduction, and possible quinidine toxicity (ventricular arrhythmias, hypotension, exacerbation of heart failure).
quinupristin	2	3	2	May result in increased risk of verapamil toxicity (dizziness, headache, flushing, peripheral edema).
ranolazine	0	1	2	May result in increased ranolazine steady-state plasma concentrations and increased risk of cardiotoxicity (QT prolongation, torsades de pointes, cardiac arrest).
rifapentine	2	3	2	May result in decreased CCB effectiveness.
ritonavir	2	3	2	May result in increased verapamil serum concentrations and potential toxicity (dizziness, headache, flushing, peripheral edema, cardiac arrhythmias).
saquinavir	1	3	2	May result in increased risk of verapamil toxicity (dizziness, headache, flushing, peripheral edema, cardiac arrhythmias).
simvastatin	2	2	2	May result in increased risk of myopathy or rhabdomyolysis.
sirolimus	0	3	1	May result in increased plasma sirolimus concentrations and risk of sirolimus toxicity.

ONSET: 0 – NOT SPECIFIED 1 – RAPID 2 – DELAYED   SEVERITY: 1 – CONTRAINDICATED 2 – MAJOR 3 – MODERATE

St. John's wort	2	3	2	May result in reduced bioavailability of verapamil.
tubocurarine	1	3	2	May result in enhanced neuromuscular blockade.
vecuronium	1	3	2	May result in enhanced neuromuscular blockade.
voriconazole	0	3	2	May result in increased plasma concentrations of CCB.

WARFARIN

acarbose	2	3	2	May result in increased risk of bleeding.
acemetacin	2	3	2	May result in increased risk of bleeding.
acetaminophen	2	3	1	May result in increased risk of bleeding.
allopurinol	2	3	2	May result in increased risk of bleeding.
aminoglutethimide	2	3	2	May result in decreased anticoagulant effectiveness.
amiodarone	2	3	2	May result in increased risk of bleeding.
amitriptyline	2	3	2	May result in increased risk of bleeding.
amoxicillin	0	3	2	May result in increased risk of bleeding.
amprenavir	2	3	2	May result in potentiation of anticoagulant effects.
Anticoagulants (*abciximab, acenocoumarol, ancrod, anisindione, antithrombin III human, bivalirudin, cilostazol, clopidogrel, danaparoid, defibrotide, dermatan sulfate, dicumarol, eptifibatide, fondaparinux, lamifiban,*	0	2	2	May result in increased risk of bleeding.

pentosan polysulfate sodium, phenindione, phenprocoumon, sibrafiban, xemilofiban)				
Antithyroid Agents (*carbimazole, methimazole, methylthiouracil, potassium iodide, propylthiouracil*)	2	3	2	May result in decreased anticoagulant effectiveness.
apazone	2	3	2	May result in increased risk of bleeding.
aprepitant	2	2	2	May result in reduced plasma concentration of warfarin, which decreases the INR or prothrombin time.
aspirin	2	2	1	May result in increased risk of bleeding.
avocado	2	3	2	May result in reduced anticoagulant effectiveness.
azathioprine	2	3	2	May result in decreased anticoagulant effectiveness.
azithromycin	2	3	2	May result in increased risk of bleeding.
benzbromarone	2	3	2	May result in increased risk of bleeding.
bosentan	2	3	2	May result in reduced warfarin efficacy.
bromfenac	2	3	2	May result in increased risk of bleeding.
butabarbital	2	3	2	May result in decreased anticoagulant effectiveness.
butalbital	2	3	2	May result in decreased anticoagulant effectiveness.
capecitabine	2	2	1	May result in increased risk of bleeding.

ONSET: 0 – NOT SPECIFIED 1 – RAPID 2 – DELAYED   SEVERITY: 1 – CONTRAINDICATED 2 – MAJOR 3 – MODERATE

carbamazepine	2	3	2	May result in decreased anticoagulant effectiveness.
cefamandole	2	3	2	May result in increased risk of bleeding.
cefazolin	2	3	2	May result in increased risk of bleeding.
celecoxib	2	2	2	May result in increased risk of bleeding.
chloral hydrate	1	3	2	May result in increased risk of bleeding.
cholestyramine	2	3	2	May result in decreased effects of warfarin.
chondroitin	2	3	2	May result in elevations of INR serum values and potentiation of anticoagulant effects.
cimetidine	2	3	2	May result in increased risk of bleeding.
ciprofloxacin	2	3	2	May result in increased risk of bleeding.
cisapride	2	3	2	May result in increased risk of bleeding.
clarithromycin	2	3	2	May result in increased risk of bleeding.
coenzyme Q10	2	3	2	May result in reduced anticoagulant effectiveness.
Contraceptives, Combination (*ethinyl estradiol, etonogestrel, levonorgestrel, mestranol, norelgestromin, norethindrone, norgestrel*)	2	3	2	May result in decreased or increased anticoagulant effectiveness.
cranberry	2	2	2	May result in increased risk of bleeding.
curcumin	2	3	2	May result in increased risk of bleeding.

cyclosporine	2	3	2	May result in decreased anticoagulant and cyclosporine effectiveness.
danazol	2	3	2	May result in increased risk of bleeding.
darunavir	2	3	2	May result in altered warfarin concentrations.
desvenlafaxine	0	2	2	May result in increased risk of bleeding.
dicloxacillin	2	3	2	May result in decreased anticoagulant effect of warfarin.
diflunisal	2	3	2	May result in increased risk of bleeding.
disopyramide	2	3	2	May result in increased risk of bleeding.
disulfiram	2	3	2	May result in increased risk of bleeding.
dong quai	2	3	2	May result in increased risk of bleeding.
doxepin	2	3	2	May result in increased risk of bleeding.
duloxetine	2	2	2	May result in increased INR and increased risk of bleeding.
enoxacin	2	3	2	May result in increased risk of bleeding.
erlotinib	2	3	2	May result in increased risk of bleeding.
erythromycin	2	3	2	May result in increased risk of bleeding.
esomeprazole	2	3	2	May result in elevations in INR serum values and potentiation of anticoagulation effects.

ONSET: 0 - NOT SPECIFIED 1 - RAPID 2 - DELAYED   SEVERITY: 1 - CONTRAINDICATED 2 - MAJOR 3 - MODERATE

eterobarb	2	3	2	May result in decreased anticoagulant effectiveness.
exenatide	0	3	2	May result in increased INR.
felbamate	2	3	2	May result in increased risk of bleeding.
fenofibrate	2	2	2	May result in increased INR and risk of bleeding events.
fluconazole	2	3	2	May result in increased risk of bleeding.
fluorouracil	2	3	1	May result in increased risk of bleeding.
fluoxetine	2	3	2	May result in increased risk of bleeding.
fluoxymesterone	2	3	2	May result in increased risk of bleeding.
fluvastatin	2	3	2	May result in increased risk of bleeding.
fluvoxamine	2	3	2	May result in increased risk of bleeding.
fosamprenavir	2	3	2	May result in increased warfarin plasma concentrations.
garlic	2	2	2	May result in increased risk of bleeding.
gefitinib	0	3	2	May result in increased risk of bleeding.
gemcitabine	1	3	2	May result in increased risk of bleeding.
gemfibrozil	2	3	2	May result in increased risk of bleeding.
ginger	2	3	2	May result in increased risk of bleeding.
ginkgo	2	2	2	May result in increased risk of bleeding.
ginseng	2	3	2	May result in decreased INR and anticoagulant effects.

glucagon	2	3	2	May result in increased risk of bleeding.
glucosamine	2	3	2	May result in elevations of INR serum values and potentiation of anticoagulant effects.
glyburide	2	3	2	May result in increased risk of bleeding.
green tea	2	3	2	May result in reduced anticoagulant effectiveness.
griseofulvin	2	3	2	May result in decreased anticoagulant effectiveness.
high-protein food	2	3	2	May result in reduced warfarin anticoagulant effectiveness.
ifosfamide	2	3	2	May result in increased risk of bleeding.
imatinib	0	2	2	May result in increased risk of bleeding.
indomethacin	2	3	2	May result in increased risk of bleeding.
indoprofen	2	3	2	May result in increased risk of bleeding.
isoniazid	2	3	2	May result in increased risk of bleeding.
isoxicam	2	3	2	May result in increased risk of bleeding.
itraconazole	2	3	2	May result in increased risk of bleeding.
ketoconazole	2	3	2	May result in increased risk of bleeding.
ketoprofen	2	2	2	May result in increased risk of bleeding.
lactulose	0	3	2	May result in elevated INR serum values with potentiation of anticoagulation effects.

ONSET: 0 = NOT SPECIFIED 1 = RAPID 2 = DELAYED   SEVERITY: 1 = CONTRAINDICATED 2 = MAJOR 3 = MODERATE

lansoprazole	2	3	2	May result in elevations in INR serum values and potentiation of anticoagulation effects.
leflunomide	2	2	2	May result in increased risk of bleeding.
lepirudin	1	3	2	May result in excessive bleeding.
levamisole	2	3	2	May result in increased risk of bleeding.
levofloxacin	2	3	2	May result in increased risk of bleeding.
lornoxicam	2	3	2	May result in increased risk of bleeding.
lycium	2	2	2	May result in increased risk of bleeding.
melatonin	2	3	2	May result in increased risk of bleeding.
meloxicam	2	3	2	May result in increased risk of bleeding.
menthol	0	3	2	May result in reduced anticoagulant effectiveness of warfarin.
mephobarbital	2	3	2	May result in decreased anticoagulant effectiveness.
mercaptopurine	2	3	2	May result in decreased anticoagulant effectiveness.
mesalamine	2	3	2	May result in decreased warfarin efficacy.
mesna	2	3	2	May result in increased risk of bleeding.
methyl salicylate	2	3	2	May result in increased risk of bleeding.
methylprednisolone	2	3	2	May result in increased risk of bleeding or diminished effects of anticoagulant.

methyltestosterone	2	3	2	May result in increased risk of bleeding.
metronidazole	2	3	2	May result in increased risk of bleeding.
miconazole	2	3	2	May result in increased risk of bleeding.
mitotane	2	3	2	May result in decreased warfarin effectiveness.
moricizine	2	3	2	May result in increased risk of bleeding.
moxifloxacin	2	2	1	May result in increased risk of bleeding.
nafcillin	2	3	2	May result in decreased anticoagulant effectiveness.
nalidixic acid	2	3	2	May result in increased risk of bleeding.
naproxen	2	2	2	May result in increased risk of bleeding.
nevirapine	2	3	2	May result in decreased warfarin effectiveness.
nilutamide	2	3	2	May result in increased risk of bleeding.
nimesulide	2	3	2	May result in increased risk of bleeding.
noni juice	2	3	2	May result in risk of acquiring warfarin resistance.
norfloxacin	2	3	2	May result in increased risk of bleeding.
ofloxacin	2	3	2	May result in increased risk of bleeding.
omeprazole	2	3	2	May result in elevations of INR serum values and potentiation of anticoagulant effects.
orlistat	0	3	2	May result in increased risk of bleeding.

ONSET: 0 = NOT SPECIFIED, 1 = RAPID, 2 = DELAYED   SEVERITY: 1 = CONTRAINDICATED, 2 = MAJOR, 3 = MODERATE

oxandrolone	2	2	2	May result in increased anticoagulant response and increased risk of bleeding.
oxyphenbutazone	2	3	2	May result in increased risk of bleeding.
pantoprazole	0	3	2	May result in increased INR and prothrombin time.
paroxetine	2	3	2	May result in increased risk of bleeding.
phenobarbital	2	3	1	May result in decreased anticoagulant effectiveness.
phenylbutazone	2	3	2	May result in increased risk of bleeding.
phytonadione	2	3	2	May result in change in or fluctuation of INR.
piracetam	2	3	2	May result in increased risk of bleeding.
primidone	2	3	2	May result in decreased anticoagulant effectiveness.
proguanil	2	2	2	May result in enhanced anticoagulant effect.
propafenone	2	3	2	May result in increased risk of bleeding.
propoxyphene	2	3	2	May result in increased risk of bleeding.
quetiapine	2	3	2	May result in potentiation of anticoagulant effects.
ranitidine	2	3	2	May result in increased risk of bleeding.
rifabutin	2	3	2	May result in reduced warfarin effectiveness.
rifapentine	2	3	2	May result in decreased anticoagulant effectiveness.
ritonavir	2	3	2	May result in decreased plasma warfarin concentrations.

rofecoxib	1	3	2	May result in increased risk of bleeding.
rosuvastatin	2	3	2	May result in increased INR and increased risk of bleeding.
roxithromycin	2	3	2	May result in increased risk of bleeding.
Salicylates (benorilate, choline salicylate, polyacrylamide, salicylamide, salicyclic acid, salsalate, sodium salicylate, sodium thiosalicylate, trolamine salicylate)	2	3	2	May result in increased risk of bleeding.
saquinavir	2	3	2	May result in increased risk of bleeding.
secobarbital	2	3	2	May result in decreased anticoagulant effectiveness.
simvastatin	2	3	1	May result in increased risk of bleeding and an increased risk of rhabdomyolysis.
soy isoflavones	2	3	2	May result in reduced warfarin effectiveness.
soy protein	2	3	2	May result in reduced warfarin effectiveness.
soybean	2	3	2	May result in reduced warfarin effectiveness.
SSRIs (citalopram, clovoxamin, femoxetine, flexinoxan, fluoxetine, fluvoxamine, nefazodone, paroxetine, sertraline, venlafaxine, zimeldine)	0	2	2	May result in increased risk of bleeding.
St. John's wort	2	2	2	May result in decreased warfarin plasma concentrations leading to reduced anticoagulant effectiveness.

ONSET: 0 - NOT SPECIFIED 1 - RAPID 2 - DELAYED   SEVERITY: 1 - CONTRAINDICATED 2 - MAJOR 3 - MODERATE

stanozolol	2	3	2	May result in increased risk of bleeding.
sucralfate	2	3	2	May result in decreased warfarin effectiveness.
sulfamethoxazole	2	2	2	May result in increased risk of bleeding.
sulfinpyrazone	2	3	2	May result in increased risk of bleeding.
sulfisoxazole	2	2	2	May result in increased risk of bleeding.
sulindac	2	3	2	May result in increased risk of bleeding.
tamoxifen	2	2	2	May result in increased risk of bleeding.
tan-shen	2	2	2	May result in increased risk of bleeding.
tenidap	2	3	2	May result in increased risk of bleeding.
terbinafine	2	3	2	May result in alteration of warfarin efficacy.
Thyroid Hormones (*dextrothyroxine, levothyroxine, liothyronine, thyroglobulin, thyroid*)	2	3	2	May result in increased risk of bleeding.
tibolone	2	3	1	May result in potentiation of warfarin-induced anticoagulation.
ticlopidine	2	3	2	May result in increased concentration of the R-warfarin enantiomer and/or increased risk of bleeding.
tolterodine	2	3	2	May result in increased risk of bleeding.
tramadol	2	3	2	May result in increased prothrombin time and an increased risk of bleeding.

trastuzumab	2	3	2	May result in increased risk of bleeding.
valdecoxib	2	3	2	May result in increased risk of bleeding.
vancomycin	2	3	2	May result in increased risk of bleeding.
venlafaxine	0	3	2	May result in increased risk of bleeding.
vitamin A	2	3	2	May result in increased risk of bleeding.
vitamin E	2	3	2	May result in increased risk of bleeding.
vitamin K-containing food	2	3	1	May result in altered anticoagulant effectiveness.
voriconazole	0	2	2	May result in potentiation of warfarin induced prothrombin time and increased risk of bleeding.
vorinostat	0	3	2	May result in increased risk of bleeding.
zafirlukast	2	3	2	May result in increased risk of bleeding.
zileuton	2	3	2	May result in significant increase in prothrombin time.
ZOLPIDEM				
bupropion	2	3	2	May result in increased risk of hallucinations.
desipramine	2	3	2	May result in increased risk of hallucinations.
ethanol	1	3	2	May result in increased sedation.
ketoconazole	1	3	2	May result in increased plasma concentrations and pharmacodynamic effects of zolpidem.

rifampin	1	3	2	May result in decreased plasma concentration and pharmacodynamic effect of zolpidem.
sertraline	2	3	2	May result in increased risk of hallucinations.
venlafaxine	2	3	2	May result in increased risk of hallucinations.